Bottom Line's

100 HOTTEST NEW NATURAL CURES AND COVER-UPS

D0840260

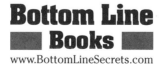

Bottom Line
Books

www.BottomLineSecrets.com

BOTTOM LINE'S HOTTEST NEW NATURAL CURES AND COVER-UPS

TABLE OF CONTENTS

BOTTOM LINE'S
HOTTEST NEW
NATURAL CURES
AND COVER-UPS

REPORT #1

A COMPLETE PLAN TO
LOWER YOUR CHOLESTEROL

Source: **Robert E. Kowalski**, medical journalist and author of *The New 8-Week Cholesterol Cure—The Ultimate Program for Preventing Heart Disease*. HarperCollins. He is editor of *The Diet-Heart Newsletter*, PO Box 2039, Venice, CA 90294. *www. thehealthyheart.net*.

Robert Kowalski has written about—and personally struggled with—high cholesterol for years. From his unique perspective, he offers the following lessons from his medical research and personal experience. **HERE'S WHAT HE HAD TO SAY...**

How is your cholesterol level these days?

I'm a shining example of how successful "secondary prevention" can be. When I left the hospital after my first bypass operation in 1978, the doctors basically told me, "We've fixed the problem—now go out and enjoy your life."

Six years later, I was back in the hospital for another bypass. That's when I started to research cholesterol and came up with the idea of controlling my cholesterol through a diet low in fat and high in oat bran—plus daily doses of the vitamin niacin.

Lo and behold, my total cholesterol dropped from 269 to 184 in only *eight weeks*. I've had angiograms since then, and today my coronary vessels are clear.

What is your advice for people at risk for heart disease?

Start by taking a daily multivitamin supplement, along with an additional 1,000 micrograms (mcg) of folic acid...6 milligrams (mg) of vitamin B-6 and 500 mcg of vitamin B-12.

These B vitamins "normalize" blood levels of *homocysteine* —an amino acid that is as much a predictor of heart attack risk as is high cholesterol.

Ask your doctor to check your cholesterol levels—including total cholesterol, LDL ("bad") cholesterol and HDL ("good") cholesterol. Make sure he/she checks your triglyceride levels, also.

These numbers indicate your risk for coronary artery disease. Regardless of your age, try to get your total cholesterol below 200 with an LDL level no higher than 100.

What if a person's total cholesterol exceeds 200?

You can lower your cholesterol level by about 10% simply by eating oat bran. When you eat one cup of oat bran (the equivalent of three bran muffins) or one-and-a-half cups of oatmeal each day, the bran binds with bile in your digestive tract. The bile is then excreted in bowel movements.

Since bile contains cholesterol, more blood cholesterol must then be used up to make additional bile. Other foods that are high in soluble fiber, such as dried beans, raisins, prunes and figs, also help eliminate bile.

What about soy foods?

Eating soy can yield another 10% drop in cholesterol, but you've got to consume a fair amount—25 grams (g) of soy protein a day. That's the equivalent of three eight-ounce glasses of soy milk, plus soy nut snacks.

NOTE: Soy is high in *phytoestrogens*, which means that some people, especially women at risk for breast cancer, may not want to consume large amounts.

If you adopt these approaches, you'll make a real dent in your cholesterol. The other step is to cut back on dietary fat.

Does this mean cutting out all fat?

No. You can eat all the fish you want, especially fatty fish, since it contains heart-protective omega-3 fatty acids. Also, use as much olive oil and canola oil as you want.

Just be sure to cut back on trans fat (referred to on food labels as "hydrogenated" or "partially hydrogenated" fat or vegetable oil). Saturated fat, too, should be limited.

Trans fat not only raises levels of total and LDL cholesterol, but also lowers levels of protective HDL cholesterol.

Another huge source of trans fat is fast-food restaurants, which fry their products in hydrogenated fat. Have fast food no more than once a week. (Never is best.)

To reduce your intake of saturated fat, substitute avocados, nuts or peanut butter for meat whenever possible. Consume skim milk instead of low-fat milk products. Remove skin from chicken. And eat only lean cuts of meat.

If you plan on eating hamburgers or meat loaf, pick out a piece of lean London broil or top round at the supermarket and ask the butcher to trim the fat before grinding it. You'll have ground beef that's only 5% fat—the same fat content as skinless chicken breast. Regular ground beef is 15% to 30% fat.

Where does niacin come into the picture?

If your cholesterol is in the mid-200s or higher, talk to your doctor about taking cholesterol-lowering medication.

I'm not a doctor, but I prefer niacin, a vitamin of the B-complex group, to statin drugs—for several reasons. First, statins are expensive, and not everyone has insurance that covers the cost. Second, we know next to nothing about the long-term side effects of statins. Finally, while statins lower LDL and total cholesterol, they don't affect HDLs, triglycerides or other cholesterol "subfractions."

Niacin lowers total and LDL cholesterol *and* triglycerides. It also raises HDL *and* lowers levels of two other dangerous particles—lipoprotein subfraction alpha, or lp(a) cholesterol, and small, dense LDL cholesterol, both of which are especially prone to lodging in artery walls.

But niacin does have a downside. You have to take it three times a day (typically one 500-mg tablet with each meal) and have your liver enzymes checked *every six months*, since the high dosage required for cholesterol reduction can cause liver disturbances. Niacin can also cause flushing.

A new therapy that combines statins and niacin is showing promise in clinical trials. In one recent study of heart patients at the University of Washington, the results of this approach virtually halted the progression of heart disease. Statin drugs alone did not.

■

REPORT #2

BLOOD-THINNERS THAT CAUSE STROKES

Source: **Rebecca Shannonhouse,** editor, *Bottom Line/Health*, 281 Tresser Blvd., Stamford, CT 06901.

When Israeli Prime Minister Ariel Sharon suffered a clot-related ischemic stroke, he received an anticoagulant drug to help prevent additional clots from forming. The following month, he suffered a hemorrhagic stroke (bleeding in the brain). Did the anticoagulant cause the second stroke? There is no definitive answer, but Sharon's case is raising new questions about the use of these powerful drugs.

BACKGROUND: Between 10% and 15% of patients who suffer an ischemic stroke will have another ischemic stroke within a year. An anticoagulant helps prevent such a recurrence in certain patients, including those with atrial fibrillation (a heart-rhythm irregularity).

However, choosing the right drug can be tricky. Every anticoagulant—including *warfarin* (Coumadin), *enoxaparin* (Lovenox) and *heparin*—has the potential to cause bleeding in the brain, explains David Chiu, MD, medical director of the Methodist Hospital Stroke Center in Houston.

If you take an anticoagulant—or one is recommended for you—here's what you should know...

• *Anticoagulants are mainly used for a heart attack*...atrial fibrillation, which can cause clots...or clots in the legs (deep-vein thrombosis) or lungs (pulmonary embolism).

• *Patients hospitalized for ischemic stroke* are sometimes treated with the injectable anticoagulant heparin or enoxaparin. But oral antiplatelet drugs, such as aspirin or *clopidogrel*

(Plavix), are often better for long-term stroke prevention because they are less likely to cause bleeding in the brain.

■

REPORT #3

THE GREATEST NEW CHOLESTEROL CURE

Source: **Kenneth H. Cooper, MD, MPH,** founder of the Cooper Aerobics Center in Dallas. A leading expert in preventive medicine and the health benefits
of exercise and cholesterol control, he is author of *Controlling Cholesterol the
Natural Way.* Bantam.

Cholesterol-lowering statin drugs are among the most
widely prescribed drugs in the United States.

Although statins are generally safe for most people, they can
cause diarrhea, muscle pain or liver damage in 2% to 10% of
patients. These drugs also cost up to $1,800 for a year's supply
and must be taken for life.

That's why I prescribe statins only when a patient's total
cholesterol is about 240 milligrams per deciliter (mg/dL) or
higher...or when a patient already has heart disease or a high
risk of developing it due to smoking, high blood pressure or
other coronary risk factors.

Drug companies don't advertise this, but many people can
lower their cholesterol without taking medication. Talk to your
doctor about the best cholesterol-lowering regimen for you.

BEST APPROACH: It's important to eat foods that have anti-
cholesterol properties. Along with basic lifestyle changes, the
right diet can effectively lower your cholesterol to safe levels.

BONUS: If you eventually need a statin drug to cut cholesterol levels even more, consuming these foods will allow you
to take the lowest possible dose.

THE DIET CURE...

Even people with moderately elevated cholesterol (above
200) should be on a low-fat diet. This means limiting total fat
calories to 30% or less of your total fat intake. Saturated fats,

found in butter, meats and baked goods, should account for no more than 10% of total calories.

However, low-fat diets are not the perfect solution. Even with such diets, cholesterol rarely drops more than 50 points, which is not enough for some people. Also, a low-fat diet reduces levels of beneficial high-density lipoprotein (HDL) cholesterol along with the harmful low-density lipoprotein (LDL).

To compensate, everyone with high cholesterol needs to eat "functional" foods daily. These are natural and laboratory-modified foods that inhibit cholesterol absorption or promote its excretion from the body. I advise patients to eat both types of these foods to get the most cholesterol-lowering benefits.

BE SURE TO EAT...

• *Traditional functional foods.* The soluble fiber in certain grains, legumes and fruits dissolves and forms a gel in the intestine. This gel traps cholesterol molecules and prevents them from being absorbed into the bloodstream. People who eat 7 to 8 grams (g) of soluble fiber daily can lower total cholesterol 5% to 8%. **BEST OPTIONS...**

• Psyllium. This ancient Indian grain is added to some breakfast cereals as well as commercial laxatives. In one study, eating as little as 3 g of psyllium daily lowered total cholesterol by 15% and LDL by 20%.

Many breakfast cereals, including Kellogg's All-Bran Bran Buds and other multigrain cereals, contain psyllium. Or you can take three tablespoons of Metamucil daily, which is equivalent to about 10 g of soluble fiber.

• Oat and rice bran. New studies show that people who eat three ounces of oat bran daily can improve the ratio of "bad" LDL to "good" HDL cholesterol by 24%.

Rice bran lowers LDL almost as much as oat bran in those who eat approximately three ounces daily.

• *Fish.* Two to three fish meals weekly will lower LDL and triglycerides, fats that have also been linked to heart disease.

One study of 20,000 American doctors found that one meal of salmon, tuna or other omega-3-rich fish per week reduced the risk for fatal heart attack by 52%.

Fish-oil supplements are an option for people who don't eat fish, but they may not provide as many health benefits as fish.

TYPICAL DOSE: 1 to 3 g daily.

• *Designed functional foods.* The trans fats in traditional margarines raise cholesterol about as much as saturated fat. *Benecol*, a brand of cholesterol-lowering margarine, contains *stanol esters*, chemically modified plant extracts that lower cholesterol as effectively as some drugs.

Eating three tablespoons of Benecol (the equivalent of three pats) daily lowers LDL by up to 14%. Benecol is also available in gel tablets for people who want the convenience of supplements or don't eat margarine.

HELPFUL: A low-calorie version, Benecol Light, contains approximately 30% fewer calories. It can be spread on toast, bagels, etc., but it should not be used for cooking. You can cook with regular Benecol, however.

ADDITIONAL STRATEGIES...

In addition to following a low-fat diet and eating functional foods, people with high cholesterol should consider...

• *Vitamins.* Certain antioxidant vitamins reduce the risk of heart attack by blocking the chemical changes (oxidation) that cause LDL cholesterol to stick to arterial walls and promote *atherosclerosis* (fatty buildup in the arteries).

• Vitamin E. Take the natural form (d-alpha-tocopherol) daily. Consult your doctor for the appropriate amount.

• Vitamin C. Like vitamin E, it inhibits oxidation of LDL molecules. People who get the most vitamin C through their diets or from supplements are less likely to die from cardiovascular disease than those who get smaller amounts.

DOSAGE: 500 mg, twice daily, in supplement form.

• *Exercise.* We used to think that only vigorous workouts would elevate levels of beneficial HDL cholesterol.

NEW RESEARCH: Walking or jogging at low to moderate intensity—for example, walking a mile in about 14 minutes—can raise HDLs by as much as 9%.

I advise my patients to walk briskly for 30 minutes at least three days a week, then after two weeks to add additional exercises, such as calisthenics and weight training.

BONUS: Combining a healthful diet with aerobic exercise can lower LDLs by up to 20 points.

• *Weight loss.* It's not clear why, but many people who lose weight also reduce their LDL cholesterol levels. Total cholesterol typically drops by about 5% for every five to 10 pounds of weight loss.

• *Niacin.* High doses of this B vitamin (1.5 to 3 g daily) can lower LDLs 15% to 30% and raise HDLs 10% to 40%.

Niacin can be taken alone, but is normally added if statins do not lower triglycerides or raise HDL sufficiently. At high doses, niacin can cause side effects, such as flushing, liver problems and heart-rhythm irregularities. Use it only under a doctor's supervision. A year's supply costs about $100.

■

REPORT #4

THE ULTIMATE CHOLESTEROL-LOWERING DIET

Source: **John McDougall, MD,** founder and medical director of the McDougall Program, Santa Rosa, CA. 800-941-7111 or *www.drmcdougall.com.* He is author of *The McDougall Program for a Healthy Heart—A Life-Saving Approach to Preventing and Treating Heart Disease.* Diane Publishing.

The importance of lowering cholesterol levels was underscored when the National Institutes of Health (NIH) released new guidelines that called for the aggressive treatment of total cholesterol levels of 240 or higher. NIH recommended aiming for a level of 200 or below.

With my patients, I go even further—I work with them to achieve and maintain a total cholesterol level *no higher than 150.* This is the point where heart disease stops progressing and begins to reverse itself. This is also a level of cholesterol where the risk of dying from heart disease is almost zero. If you settle for a total cholesterol of 200 instead, you still subject your arteries to toxins and plaque buildup—and risk a heart attack.

Here's how I help my high-cholesterol patients get their levels under control...

CUT OUT ANIMAL PRODUCTS...

The single most effective way to lower your blood cholesterol is to stop eating foods that contain cholesterol. In other words, *avoid all animal products*—red meat, poultry, shellfish, fish, eggs, dairy products and foods made with them.

As far as the health of your arteries is concerned, there is no "safe" amount of animal products.

Forbidden foods (many of which have long been perceived as permissible) include...

• *Fish and fowl.* Studies show these foods will raise cholesterol just as surely as beef or pork.

• *Low-fat or skim milk, cheese or other dairy products.* Even when the fat is taken out, the animal proteins in these foods can raise cholesterol levels and damage the artery walls.

• *"Free" fats such as margarine, corn oil, olive oil and canola oil.* These fats are easily oxidized in the bloodstream, making plaque likely to build up on artery walls.

If you follow a strict vegetarian diet for several months, you can lower your cholesterol levels by 25% or more. At the same time, blood levels of triglycerides, homocysteine, uric acid and other heart disease risk factors will also decline.

VEGETARIAN DELIGHTS...

Giving up animal products does not mean you must eat poorly. The foods in my program are varied and delicious. They provide all needed nutrients in optimal amounts.

You can eat *all you want* of the following...

• *Whole grains, including barley, brown rice, buckwheat, bulgur, corn, oatmeal and wheat,* as well as noodles made from these sources.

• *Potatoes, sweet potatoes and yams.*

• *Root vegetables,* such as beets, carrots and turnips.

• *Squashes,* such as acorn, buttercup and zucchini squash.

• *Beans and peas,* including chickpeas, green peas, kidney beans, lentils and string beans.

• *Other vegetables,* such as broccoli, brussels sprouts, cabbage, celery, dark lettuce, spinach, cucumber, okra, onions, peppers and mushrooms.

• *Mild spices and cooking herbs.*

Eat only limited amounts of fruit and fruit juice (no more than three servings a day), sugar and other sweeteners, salt and fatty plant foods, such as peanut butter, seed spreads, avocados, olives and soybean products—including tofu. Simple sugars, even fruit and juice, raise cholesterol and triglycerides.

HEART-HEALTHY MENU PLAN...

There are plenty of excellent vegetarian cookbooks, but you don't have to be a gourmet to prepare heart-healthful meals. Start with potatoes, rice, beans or spaghetti, then add low-fat, plant-based sauces and soups. Throw in a salad and bread, and you've got a meal. OTHER TIPS...

• *For breakfast, toast, bagels, oatmeal, cereals, hash browns and pancakes* (all made from the right ingredients) are all fine. Use rice milk or soy milk on cold cereal.

• *Sauté food in soy sauce, wine or sherry, vinegar, vegetarian Worcestershire sauce, salsa or lemon or lime juice.*

• *Eat until you're satisfied*...and eat as often as you need to.

• *To boost feelings of fullness, include beans and peas in meals.* A typical day's menu might include...

BREAKFAST: Pancakes, oatmeal, French toast or a tortilla.

LUNCH: Vegetable soup, along with a vegetarian sandwich or a veggie burger.

DINNER: Bean burritos, mu-shu vegetables over rice, chili and rice or spaghetti with marinara sauce, along with fresh bread and a chickpea salad.

After a week or two on this diet, most people start to crave healthful foods—without all that excess dietary fat.

CHOLESTEROL-LOWERING DRUGS...

With a high-risk patient—someone who's had a heart attack or appears headed for a heart attack, coronary bypass or angio-plasty—I would not wait several months to "see what happens." If his/her total cholesterol hasn't fallen to 150 after 10 days of healthful eating, I suggest supplementing the diet with drugs.

Between a vegetarian diet and cholesterol-lowering medication, virtually anyone's cholesterol can be brought down to 150.

First, try some natural cholesterol-lowering "medications"...

• *Garlic*—up to 800 milligrams (mg), or one clove a day.

• *Oat bran*—two ounces a day, or oatmeal—three ounces, dry weight, a day.

• *Vitamin C*—2,000 mg a day.

• *Vitamin E*—dry form, consult your doctor for the appropriate amount.

• *Beta-carotene*—25,000 international units (IU) a day.

• *Gugulipid.* Recently, I've been recommending this Indian herb—500 to 1,500 mg, three times a day.

• *Immediate-release niacin* is another potentially useful medication. It can damage the liver, so it should be taken only under a doctor's supervision.

If the patient doesn't respond, I typically prescribe *simvastatin* (Zocor), *pravastatin* (Pravachol), *lovastatin* (Mevacor) or *fluvastatin* (Lescol). Since my patient may have to take this medication for years, it's important to match him with the drug that's most effective, but has the fewest side effects.

EXERCISE AND GOOD HABITS...

While exercise isn't as crucial as diet, a brisk walk of 20 minutes or more each day benefits your heart in many ways.

Regular exercise trains the heart to beat more efficiently... increases levels of HDL ("good") cholesterol...lowers levels of triglycerides...increases the flow of oxygen to your heart, brain, muscles and other tissues...and boosts the immune system.

AS IF YOU DIDN'T KNOW: Don't smoke. Limit coffee consumption (both regular and decaffeinated raise cholesterol levels about 10%). Drink alcohol moderately if at all. Your arteries will thank you.

■

REPORT #5

ARTERY BLOCKAGE DISSOLVED IN HOURS

Source: **James F. Benenati, MD,** medical director, Peripheral Vascular Laboratory, Baptist Cardiac & Vascular Institute, Miami, FL.

D angerous blood clots can be eliminated with a new ultrasound device. The device consists of a hair-thin wire with transducers attached. After it is positioned near a clot, the transducers emit a high-frequency sound to loosen blood fibers and force an anticlotting drug through the clot. The device is in limited use for people who have deep-vein thrombosis or arterial-bypass grafts in the leg or acute blood clots in leg arteries. It is being studied for more uses, including dissolving stroke-causing clots in the brain.

■

REPORT #6

GREAT GRAPE EXTRACT MAKES BLOOD PRESSURE PLUMMET

Source: **C. Tissa Kappagoda, MD, PhD,** professor of cardiovascular medicine, University of California, Davis.

Grape seed extract lowers blood pressure. In a new study, 24 patients with metabolic syndrome (a cluster of heart disease risk factors, including high blood pressure, excess abdominal weight and elevated blood sugar) took a 150 or 300 milligram (mg) capsule of grape seed extract or a placebo daily for one month.

RESULT: Those who took either dose of the extract experienced an average drop in systolic pressure (top number) of 12 millimeters of mercury (mmHg) and 8 mmHg in diastolic pressure (bottom number).

THEORY: Grape seed extract boosts the production of nitric oxide, a heart-protective enzyme. If you have prehypertension (120–139 systolic and 80–89 diastolic), ask your doctor about trying grape seed extract.

■

REPORT #7

JUICE YOUR WAY TO LOWER CHOLESTEROL

Source: **Michael T. Murray, ND,** faculty member in the department of botanical medicine at Bastyr University in Seattle. He is author of *The Complete Book of Juicing* (Three Rivers). He has also written more than 20 other books, including *Dr. Murray's Total Body Tune-Up* (Bantam). *www.doctormurray.com.*

If you find it difficult to get at least five servings of fruits and vegetables daily, fresh juices can be a convenient alternative.

Juices don't provide the same fiber content found in fruits and vegetables, but they do offer a concentrated dose of the same nutrients and phytochemicals.

EXAMPLE: To get enough beta-carotene to reduce your risk for cancer, you could eat six large carrots a day...or consume the equivalent in carrot juice—one eight-ounce glass.

NUTRITIONAL ADVANTAGES...

Fruit and vegetable juices provide high levels of antioxidants. These natural plant compounds help protect the body against cancer, heart disease, aging and other degenerative conditions.

Fresh juices are a rich source of the following antioxidants...

• *Carotenes.* Researchers have identified more than 400 carotenes, including the well-known beta-carotene.

The higher the dietary intake of carotene, the lower the risk for cancer, particularly malignancies of the lung, skin and colon.

Juicing ruptures the fruits' cell walls, releasing carotenes for easier absorption. That's why fresh juice is a richer source of carotenes than are supplements or even carotene-rich foods.

BEST CAROTENE-RICH JUICE: One beet, including the top... one-half of a medium-sized sweet potato, cut into strips...and three carrots. Juice the beet first, then the sweet potato strips and then the carrots.

• *Flavonoids function as biological stress modifiers,* altering the body's reaction to allergens, viruses and carcinogens.

The flavonoids *anthocyanidins* and *proanthocyanidins* can be found in blueberries, blackberries, cherries and grapes. These compounds increase vitamin C levels within the cells, strengthen small blood vessels and reinforce joints.

They also help prevent arthritis and hardening of the arteries (atherosclerosis), which leads to heart disease and stroke.

Other flavonoids are antiallergenic, inhibiting the formation and secretion of histamine and other inflammatory compounds that produce the allergic response.

BEST FLAVONOID-RICH JUICE: One-half cup each of blackberries, blueberries and strawberries. Plus one sliced apple or pear.

• *Chlorophyll,* the green pigment found in plants, possesses significant antioxidant and anticancer properties.

BEST CHLOROPHYLL-RICH JUICE: Four celery ribs, one-half cucumber (peeled if waxed) and one-half cup of parsley.

When preparing chlorophyll-rich juice, limit your use of greens, such as kale, lettuce or spinach, to one-fourth of the mixture. Otherwise, the juice may taste too "strong."

WHEN TO JUICE...

To add juice to your daily diet, try substituting it for your morning coffee. Or fill a thermos with juice and take it to work with you for a midmorning or midafternoon pick-me-up.

At lunch or dinner, start your meal with juice. Studies have shown that the act of drinking juice before a meal reduces your appetite.

CAUTION: Fruit and vegetable juices contain simple sugars, which should be consumed in moderation, especially if you are diabetic or hypoglycemic.

Limit your intake of fruit juice, which is particularly rich in simple sugars and calories, to one eight-ounce glass a day.

Your total intake of fruit and vegetable juice should not exceed 16 ounces a day.

■

REPORT #8

THE GRAPEFRUIT CURE FOR CHOLESTEROL

Source: **Shela Gorinstein, PhD,** chief scientist, Hebrew University of Jerusalem.

Grapefruit lowers cholesterol. In a new study, men and women whose elevated cholesterol levels did not respond to cholesterol-lowering drugs ate balanced meals with one red grapefruit, one white grapefruit or no grapefruit daily.

RESULT: Total cholesterol dropped by 15.5% in those who ate red grapefruit and by 7.6% in the white grapefruit group. Cholesterol did not drop in those who did not eat grapefruit. Grapefruit juice also may confer this benefit.

THEORY: The antioxidants that are found in grapefruit lower cholesterol levels.

CAUTION: Grapefruit can interact with some drugs. Consult your doctor.

■

REPORT #9

THE NEW "GARLIC CURE" FOR BLOCKED ARTERIES

Source: **Mark Blumenthal,** founder and executive director of the American Botanical Council (ABC), *www.herbalgram.org,* an Austin, TX-based independent, nonprofit organization dedicated to disseminating reliable information about herbs and medicinal plants. He is senior editor of the English translation of *The Complete German Commission E Monographs—Therapeutic Guide to Herbal Medicines* (Lippincott Williams & Wilkins), a clinical guide on the safety and efficacy of herbal medicines, and senior editor of *The ABC Clinical Guide to Herbs* (ABC).

It was headline news when *The New England Journal of Medicine* published a study that cast doubt on the effectiveness of echinacea. The message to the countless consumers spending more than $300 million annually on the purported cold-fighting herb? *Save your money.*

University of Virginia School of Medicine researchers had found echinacea to be no more effective than a placebo at combating cold and flu symptoms. But don't clear out your herbal medicine chest just yet.

What went largely unreported was that study participants received only 900 milligrams (mg) of echinacea daily—less than one-third of the dose recommended by the World Health Organization for combating upper-respiratory infections. That's akin to expecting one-third of a dose of aspirin to relieve a headache.

What's the other side of the story? Dozens of clinical studies point to echinacea's effectiveness, including an August 2004 Canadian trial in which volunteers who took echinacea at the onset of colds experienced 23% milder, shorter symptoms, such as sore throat, stuffy nose, chills and headache, than those taking a placebo—a benefit that researchers linked to a marked increase in circulating white blood cells and other cells of the immune system.

More work is needed to identify the optimal echinacea species (supplements are commonly derived from *E. purpurea, E. pallida* or *E. augustifolia*) and the most potent plant parts (roots, stems, leaves or flowers).

Meanwhile, best results have been achieved by taking 3,000 mg daily of an echinacea product that combines one of the above-mentioned species and parts at the first sign of cold or flu until symptoms resolve.

CAUTION: If you're allergic to ragweed, avoid echinacea supplements derived from stems, leaves or flowers—they may contain pollen and trigger a reaction. Use an echinacea root supplement.

Five other herbs with scientific evidence on their side...

GARLIC...

WHAT IT DOES: Helps prevent and possibly reverse arterial plaque buildup (atherosclerosis), a major risk factor for heart attack and stroke...reduces risk for stomach and colorectal cancers...and acts as a blood thinner to reduce the risk for blood clots.

SCIENTIFIC EVIDENCE: In a German study, 152 patients with advanced atherosclerosis who took 900 mg daily of garlic powder for four years experienced a 3% decrease in existing arterial plaques in their neck (carotid) and thigh (femoral) arteries. Those taking a placebo experienced more than a 15% *increase* in arterial plaques.

POTENTIAL SIDE EFFECTS: Bad breath and indigestion. Because garlic has a blood-thinning effect, it should not be used if you take aspirin regularly or an anticoagulant drug, such as *warfarin* (Coumadin). To minimize bleeding risk, ask your doctor about discontinuing garlic supplements at least one week before undergoing elective surgery.

TYPICAL DOSE: One clove of fresh, minced garlic daily, or 200 to 300 mg of standardized garlic powder, taken in pill or tablet form, three times daily.

GINKGO...

WHAT IT DOES: Improves memory and concentration in people with early-stage senile dementia or Alzheimer's disease, as well as in healthy adults, by increasing blood flow to the brain. May also relieve tinnitus (ringing in the ears), vertigo and altitude sickness, as well as vascular problems such as intermittent claudication, a painful calf condition caused by decreased circulation to the legs.

SCIENTIFIC EVIDENCE: An overwhelming majority of ginkgo trials have shown positive results. At least 33 randomized, controlled trials have shown this herb to enhance mental functioning or slow cognitive deterioration in older patients with dementia, while another 13 controlled studies have shown ginkgo to boost memory and cognitive performance in healthy adults.

POTENTIAL SIDE EFFECTS: Stomach upset, headache, rash and/or dizziness. Like garlic, ginkgo should not be taken with aspirin or a prescription blood thinner such as warfarin. The herb was previously believed to increase the effects of mono-amine oxidase inhibitor (MAOI) antidepressants, such as *phenelzine* (Nardil), but this has been refuted.

TYPICAL DOSE: 120 mg daily. Nearly all positive ginkgo trials have used one of three formulations that are produced in Germany and sold in health-food stores in the US under the brand names Ginkoba by Pharmaton Natural Health Products...Ginkgold by Nature's Way...and Ginkai by Abkit Inc.

MILK THISTLE...

WHAT IT DOES: Because of its strong antioxidant activity, milk thistle detoxifies the liver and may help regenerate liver cells. It may be appropriate for patients with alcohol-related liver damage or infectious or drug-induced hepatitis, as well as anyone who is regularly exposed to industrial pollutants.

SCIENTIFIC EVIDENCE: At least 19 out of 21 clinical studies (a total of 2,200 people out of 2,400) have shown milk thistle to protect the liver against invasive toxins and possibly even stimulate the generation of new liver cells.

POTENTIAL SIDE EFFECT: Loose stools.

TYPICAL DOSE: Take 140 mg of milk thistle three times daily.

SAW PALMETTO...

WHAT IT DOES: Relieves the symptoms of benign prostatic hyperplasia (BPH), a noncancerous swelling of the prostate gland, which causes frequent and/or weak urination and is common in men over age 50.

SCIENTIFIC EVIDENCE: In nearly two dozen clinical trials, saw palmetto has proven almost equal to prescription drugs, such as *finasteride* (Proscar) and *terazosin* (Hytrin), for relieving the symptoms of BPH. Unlike prescription prostate medications, which can cause side effects, including diminished libido, saw palmetto causes only minor adverse effects. Saw palmetto does not inhibit the production of prostate specific antigen (PSA), a protein that, when elevated, serves as an early warning for prostate cancer. (Conventional BPH drugs suppress PSA, complicating prostate cancer screening.)

POTENTIAL SIDE EFFECTS: Stomach upset or nausea if taken on an empty stomach.

TYPICAL DOSE: 320 mg daily. It requires four to six weeks to take effect.

VALERIAN...

WHAT IT DOES: The root combats insomnia and acts as a mild sedative to relieve anxiety or restlessness.

SCIENTIFIC EVIDENCE: All of the nearly 30 clinical studies to date have shown the herb to be effective against insomnia and anxiety. In a recent German trial, taking 600 mg of valerian root extract daily proved as effective as the prescription tranquilizer *oxazepam* (Serax) for improving sleep quality, but with fewer side effects. Unlike prescription sleep aids, valerian isn't habit-forming, won't leave you feeling groggy the next morning and doesn't diminish alertness, reaction time or concentration.

POTENTIAL SIDE EFFECTS: None known. It is best to avoid combining valerian with conventional sedatives, such as *diazepam* (Valium), since the herb may exacerbate the drug's sedating effects.

TYPICAL DOSE: 2 to 3 g of the dried crushed root, infused as a tea...or 400 to 800 mg in supplement form, taken one-half hour before bedtime.

■

REPORT #10

HEAL YOUR HEART WITH GRAPE JUICE

Source: **John Folts, PhD,** professor of medicine, University of Wisconsin Medical School, Madison.

Purple grape juice prevents dangerous blood clots even more effectively than aspirin. *Flavonoids* in the juice reduce platelet "stickiness" by about 40%. Researchers believe the same benefits can be derived from red wine and other kinds of grape juice—but not from grapes or "grape drink," which isn't 100% juice. The clot-fighting properties of grape juice are especially beneficial for certain heart patients.

■

REPORT #11

HIBISCUS FOR YOUR HEART

Source: Journal of the Science of Food and Agriculture news release.

Hibiscus flowers may help your heart in the same way as red wine and tea—with antioxidants that help control cholesterol levels and reduce heart disease, according to Chinese researchers.

They found that rats fed a hibiscus flower extract had significantly reduced cholesterol levels in their blood.

"Experiments have shown that compounds extracted from red wine and tea reduce cholesterol and lipid buildup in the arteries of rats," says lead researcher Chau-Jong Wang, of Chung Shan Medical University in Taiwan. "This is the first study to show that hibiscus extract has the same effect."

Hibiscus is used in folk medicine to treat hypertension and liver disorders.

■

REPORT #12

NUTS VS. CHOLESTEROL

Source: **Wanda Morgan, PhD, RD,** associate professor of human nutrition and food science, New Mexico State University, Las Cruces.

Eating moderate amounts of pecans (three-quarters of a cup daily for eight weeks) can lower LDL ("bad") cholesterol levels by 10%, a recent study has shown.

The monounsaturated and polyunsaturated fats in the nuts are responsible for this effect, especially when nuts take the place of saturated fats in the diet.

Studies with almonds and walnuts have shown similar results. Nuts are also high in heart-healthy fiber, vitamin E, copper and magnesium.

■

REPORT #13

ALMONDS CUT CHOLESTEROL

Source: **Gene Spiller, PhD,** director, Health Research and Studies Center, Los Altos, CA.

In a recent study, 45 people with high cholesterol levels were placed on a diet rich in almonds, olive oil or dairy products.

RESULT: After four weeks, the almond group had LDL ("bad") cholesterol levels an average of 16 points lower than the olive oil group...and 33 points lower than the dairy group. Almonds are rich sources of monounsaturated fats, fiber and the amino acid arginine. Each of these contributes to the cholesterol-lowering effect. Even if you are taking cholesterol-lowering medication, consider including almonds in your diet...along with fruits, vegetables, beans, soy foods, whole grains and garlic.

■

REPORT #14

STRESS TESTS ARE NOT FOOLPROOF

Source: **Mehmet C. Oz, MD,** director, Cardiovascular Institute, NewYork-Presbyterian Hospital–Columbia University, New York City. He is coauthor of *You: The Owner's Manual.* HarperCollins.

Signs of heart disease can be missed by exercise stress tests. An exercise stress test, which consists of an electrocardiogram (ECG) and blood pressure measurement while exercising on a treadmill, is commonly used to identify heart problems. However, stress tests fail to identify high risk for heart attack in 25% of patients.

SELF-DEFENSE: To increase accuracy to 90%, ask your doctor also to perform a thallium scan and echocardiogram.

■

REPORT #15

THE ASTONISHING CHINESE POUND-PEELER

Source: **Robert Rosati, MD,** director of the Rice Diet Clinic and associate professor emeritus of medicine at Duke University School of Medicine in Durham, NC. He is a fellow of the American College of Physicians and the American College of Cardiology, and author, with his wife, Kitty Gurkin Rosati, MS, RD, of *The Rice Diet Solution.* Simon & Schuster. *www.ricediet.com.*

Every few years, a new "breakthrough" diet hits the bestseller lists. Millions of Americans jump on the bandwagon and hope that this time they'll lose those stubborn pounds for good. Most are disappointed.

The Rice Diet, developed more than 60 years ago, is still one of the most effective weight-loss plans. German-born Duke University physician Walter Kempner, MD, designed the diet, in which participants ate mostly rice and fruit, to treat high blood pressure. He noticed that participants not only lowered their blood pressure but also lost considerable amounts of weight—and the Rice Diet was born.

Rice and other grains play a prominent role in the diet because they're filling and low-fat. Obese men on the program at our clinic lose an average of 30 pounds in the first four weeks...obese women lose an average of 19 pounds. Most people lose between one-third and one-half pound per day over a period of months.

The Rice Diet significantly lowers blood pressure and cholesterol. People who follow it for one month have an average drop in LDL ("bad") cholesterol of 13% and a drop in blood pressure of at least 5%.

HOW IT WORKS...

There are no shortcuts to weight loss. The amount of calories expended must exceed the calories consumed. This is true of all diets, including the Atkins and Zone plans. People who follow the Rice Diet start off eating between 800 and 1,000 calories daily. That amount is gradually increased to 1,000 to 1,200 calories daily—enough for dieters to feel satisfied but still lose weight. Once people reach their desired weights, they can increase calories slightly to maintain their weight. **OTHER KEY PRINCIPLES...**

• *Sodium restriction.* The Rice Diet limits daily sodium intake to between 300 and 1,000 milligrams (mg). (The average American consumes 4,000 to 7,000 mg.) Salt stimulates the appetite. People learn to crave salt and will keep eating to get more, even when they're already full. When most salt is eliminated from the diet—in the form of snacks, processed foods, etc.— people naturally take in fewer calories.

BONUS: Restricting sodium can lower blood pressure by at least five to 10 points in some people. When salt restriction is combined with a low-fat, healthful diet, most people can lower blood pressure by 20 points or more. That's often enough to avoid medication.

• *Healthful carbohydrates.* The diet features high-fiber carbohydrates. Unlike processed carbohydrates, such as white bread, high-fiber carbs are absorbed slowly into the blood. They don't produce surges in insulin that promote weight gain. Most days, you can have seven servings of whole grains/beans, six of vegetables and three of fruits.

SERVING SIZES: Brown rice* or beans (one-third cup cooked), whole-wheat bread (one slice), pasta (one-half cup cooked), whole-grain cereals (up to one cup), fruits (one medium fruit or one cup cut fruit) and vegetables (one-half cup cooked or one cup raw).

• *Limited fat.* Because most calories in the Rice Diet come from whole grains, fruits and vegetables, fat intake is limited to between 10% and 20% of total calories. Studies show that reducing dietary fat is essential to lasting weight loss. Most dietary fat should come in the form of omega-3s (found in fish and flaxseed) or the monounsaturated fat in olive oil. Avoid or eat very small amounts of butter and full-fat dairy.

• *Limited protein.* Although protein is necessary, too much can be harmful. Scientific evidence links animal protein and the

*The Chinese call unprocessed rice *tsao mi.*

accompanying saturated fat and cholesterol with heart disease and other illnesses. The Rice Diet provides ample protein daily in the form of grains, beans, nonfat dairy, vegetables, etc.

• *Mindful eating.* Most excess calories come from unconscious eating—snacking while watching TV, eating meals while driving or eating so quickly that we're not aware of what we're tasting.

Mindful eating means chewing food slowly and paying attention to tastes and textures. People who give eating their full attention are less likely to take in more calories than they really need.

PHASE 1: DETOX...

The Rice Diet has three phases. The detox stage of the diet lasts for one week. It is designed to shed excess water weight, sodium and toxins from the body. People with food sensitivities or allergies may experience headaches, joint stiffness or other symptoms as their bodies detoxify. The discomfort rarely lasts more than a few days.

On the first day of Phase 1, you're allowed only six servings of whole grains and six servings of fruits. For the remaining six days, the diet expands to include beans, vegetables and a small amount of dairy. Each day, drink 40 to 72 ounces of liquid, preferably water.

Sample menu for days two through seven...

BREAKFAST: One-half cup whole-grain cereal or one slice of whole-wheat toast...one cup of nonfat milk or yogurt...one piece of fruit.

LUNCH: One cup cooked brown rice and/or beans or one and one-half cups of a cooked grain (such as oats or barley), starchy vegetable (such as potatoes or corn) or pasta...three cups raw vegetable salad or one and one-half cups of cooked broccoli...one cup fresh fruit salad.

DINNER: One cup cooked brown rice and/or beans or one and one-half cups of another cooked grain, starchy vegetable or pasta...three cups raw cabbage...one cup berries.

PHASE 2: WEIGHT LOSS...

This is the long-term part of the diet. You stay in Phase 2 until you reach your target. Continue to set aside one day per week for the basic rice-and-fruit diet, followed by five days of grains, beans, fruit, vegetables and nonfat dairy. One day of the week, add a serving of fish or lean meat. During Phase 2, most people lose an average of three and one-half pounds per week.

SAMPLE MENU...

BREAKFAST: One-half cup whole-grain cereal or one slice of whole-wheat toast...one cup nonfat milk...one cup fresh berries...one tablespoon dried cherries or one tablespoon all-fruit jam.

LUNCH: One cup cooked rice and/or beans, or one and one-half cups of another cooked grain, starchy vegetable or pasta... two cups spinach...one-half cup steamed broccoli or one cup raw carrots...one cup melon or fresh strawberries.

DINNER: Two-thirds cup brown rice...one-third cup beans... one cup raw spinach...one cup steamed broccoli...and one cup fresh fruit salad.

PHASE 3: MAINTENANCE...

Once you reach your target, move into the third phase of the diet. Phase 3 includes the same foods as Phase 2, but two days a week, you can enjoy another three ounces of fish or lean meat or another 200 calories of other types of foods, such as eggs, nuts and tofu. If you start to gain weight, cut back on the "extras."

∎

REPORT #16

FIBER TO THE RESCUE

Source: **David J.A. Jenkins, MD, PhD, DSc,** director, Clinical Nutrition and Risk Factor Modification Centre, St. Michael's Hospital, Toronto.

A high-fiber diet can lower cholesterol just as effectively as cholesterol-lowering statin drugs.

NEW FINDING: After only one week, total cholesterol levels dropped by at least 20% in people who consumed 100 grams of fiber daily from fruit, vegetables and nuts. Their LDL ("bad") cholesterol levels dropped by 30%. However, it is difficult to consume this much fiber each day. It may be useful to modify this diet as part of an overall cholesterol-lowering program.

IF YOU HAVE HIGH CHOLESTEROL: Talk to your doctor about eating a diet that is high in dietary fiber.

■

REPORT #17

EAT RYE BREAD FOR BETTER HEALTH

Source: **Soile Gråsten, MSc, RD,** researcher, department of clinical nutrition, University of Kuopio, Finland.

Rye bread reduces levels of bile acids linked to colon cancer. Volunteers who ate four-and-a-half slices of whole-grain rye every day for four weeks lowered their acid levels by 26%.

TRAP: Most rye bread is made with refined wheat flour, which does not offer the same health benefits. Look for bread with *whole rye flour* or *whole rye meal* listed in the ingredients ...or make your own.

■

REPORT #18

DIABETES SECRET: "SLEEP IT OFF!"

Source: **Daniel J. Gottlieb, MD, MPH,** associate professor of medicine, Boston University School of Medicine.

A recent study reported that diabetes was 151% more common in men and women who slept five hours or less per night and 79% more common in those who slept nine or more hours per night, compared with those who got seven to eight hours of sleep nightly.

THEORY: Too little—or too much—sleep impairs glucose (blood sugar) metabolism.

SELF-DEFENSE: For adequate rest, most adults need seven to eight hours of sleep per night.

■

REPORT #19

THE "APPLE CIDER VINEGAR CURE" FOR DIABETES

Source: **Mark A. Stengler, ND,** naturopathic physician in private practice, La Jolla, CA...associate clinical professor at the National College of Naturopathic Medicine, Portland, OR...author of numerous books, including *The Natural Physician's Healing Therapies* and coauthor of *Prescription for Natural Cures* (both from Bottom Line Books)...and author of the *Bottom Line/Natural Healing* newsletter.

Patients often tell me that apple cider vinegar has helped them with a variety of ailments. This intrigued me because, until recently, there was little research to back up these claims.

CURE-ALL?...

Apple cider vinegar has been singled out as beneficial for a variety of conditions, including leg cramps, stomach upset, sore throat, sinus problems, high blood pressure, obesity, osteoporosis and arthritis. It also has been used to help rid the body of toxins, improve concentration, slow aging, reduce cholesterol and fight infection.

It is used topically to treat acne, sunburn, shingles and insect bites...as a skin toner...and to prevent dandruff. Many women add it to bathwater to treat vaginitis. Two of its most common uses are for weight loss and arthritis.

THE SCIENTIFIC EVIDENCE...

Recent studies have found that consuming apple cider vinegar can improve insulin resistance, a condition in which muscle, fat and liver cells have become resistant to the uptake of the hormone *insulin* and the blood sugar *glucose* needed to provide fuel for energy.

This is common among people who have diabetes as well as in some people we consider prediabetic—that is, their blood glucose and insulin levels are approaching the numbers that define diabetes. People with insulin resistance are more likely to be overweight and have increased cholesterol and triglyceride levels as well as high blood pressure.

A 2004 study at the University of Arizona examined the effects of apple cider vinegar on 29 participants (10 had type 2 diabetes, 11 had signs that they could become diabetic and eight were healthy but "insulin sensitive"). All participants fasted and were randomly asked to drink either a vinegar solution (two tablespoons or 20 grams (g) of apple cider vinegar, some water and a bit of saccharin for flavor) or a placebo drink. The drinks were followed by a high-carbohydrate meal of one white bagel, butter and orange juice.

Researchers found that postmeal spikes of insulin and glucose in the vinegar group were significantly lower in those who had insulin resistance and slightly lower in those who had diabetes, compared with those in the placebo group. Other research has shown that apple cider vinegar helps control insulin and glucose spikes in healthy people.

HOW IT WORKS...

Researchers theorize that the *acetic acid* in any vinegar, including apple cider vinegar, interferes with the enzymes that digest carbohydrates, so carbs pass through the digestive tract without being absorbed. Acetic acid also has been shown to affect enzymes that alter glucose metabolism in liver and muscle cells, reducing insulin spikes.

Because high levels of insulin promote inflammation, taking vinegar to maintain better insulin levels will control any inflammatory response in the body. This may explain why vinegar eases arthritis pain.

DOSAGE...

People can try apple cider vinegar for weight loss, blood sugar balance and other traditional uses, including arthritis relief. Dilute one to two tablespoons (some people use as little as two teaspoons to start with) in an equal amount of water, and drink it at the beginning of a meal.

Sometimes it is more convenient to take it in supplement form. A good product is Apple Cider Vinegar Plus, which is made by Indiana Botanic Gardens (800-644-8327, *www.botanicchoice. com*). Take one capsule with each meal for a total of three capsules a day. Ninety capsules cost $25.

Apple cider vinegar can cause digestive upset in some people. If you have active ulcers, use caution when taking apple cider vinegar.

■

REPORT #20

THE HIDDEN HEALING POWER OF VINEGAR

Source: **Jamison Starbuck, ND,** naturopathic physician in family practice and a lecturer at the University of Montana, both in Missoula. She is a past president of the American Association of Naturopathic Physicians and a contributing editor to *The Alternative Advisor: The Complete Guide to Natural Therapies and Alternative Treatments.* Time-Life.

For thousands of years, vinegar has held distinction as a medicinal, culinary and household aid. In 400 BC, Hippocrates recommended drinking a vinegar solution to reduce symptoms of the common cold. "Thieves' vinegar" is reputed to date from the 14th century, when thieves would wash with vinegar to protect themselves from the Plague when robbing the homes of helpless sufferers. In America, vinegar has been used since the time of the Revolutionary War to clean wounds.

More recently, vinegar is making a comeback as a medical treatment and a gourmet culinary specialty. Proponents tout vinegar as a cure for all types of ailments, including life-threatening conditions, such as cancer, high blood pressure, kidney disease and asthma. Although these claims are false, vinegar is, in fact, a very useful natural medicine. **BECAUSE IT'S SAFE, INEXPENSIVE AND READILY AVAILABLE, VINEGAR IS WORTH TRYING FOR THE FOLLOWING CONDITIONS...**

• *Arthritis.* There's no scientific evidence, but anecdotal accounts do support the use of an apple-cider vinegar solution to help relieve arthritis pain. Drink a glass of water with two teaspoons of apple-cider vinegar and two teaspoons of honey three times a day.

• *Foot odor.* To kill odor-causing bacteria, soak feet in a solution of one part vinegar (any type) and four parts hot water nightly for 15 minutes for one week. The feet should be immersed up to the ankles. Rinse with cold water at the end of the soak. Repeat this routine as it is needed.

• *Fungal infections.* Men with jock itch (a red, itching, burning rash in the groin area) will find relief by applying a mild vinegar solution one or two times daily. Make up a solution of two tablespoons of white vinegar to 12 ounces warm water...pour it over the whole groin area at the end of a shower. Do not rinse off...simply blot dry. Five days of this treatment should be adequate. For other fungal infections, such as athlete's foot or mild nail fungus, soak the affected body part in the same type of solution used for jock itch for five minutes daily until the infection is gone.

• *Leg cramps and osteoporosis.* In both women and men, these conditions generally are caused by poor dietary absorption of minerals. To help, add one teaspoon of any type of vinegar to four ounces of water and drink during each meal. As an alternative, simply eat a salad with a vinegar-based dressing whenever you can. Vinegar's acidity will help your digestive tract to draw minerals from your food and make them more available for absorption into your bloodstream.

• *Vaginitis.* Women with bacterial or yeast vaginitis respond well and quickly to treatment with vinegar. Douche with a vinegar-and-water solution two times per day for up to five days. Purchase Massengill's premixed plain vinegar douching solution in disposable bottles. Or you can douche with your own solution, using one tablespoon white vinegar per six ounces warm water.

■

REPORT #21

REDUCE DIABETIC NERVE PAIN

Source: **Mark A. Stengler, ND,** naturopathic physician in private practice, La Jolla, CA...associate clinical professor at the National College of Naturopathic Medicine, Portland, OR...author of numerous books, including *The Natural Physician's Healing Therapies* and coauthor of *Prescription for Natural Cures* (both from Bottom Line Books)...and author of the *Bottom Line/Natural Healing* newsletter.

Researchers evaluated the effects of the nutritional supplement acetyl-L-carnitine (ALC) on diabetic neuropathy, a condition that occurs when diabetes damages the nerves, especially those in the hands, legs and feet. Symptoms include numbness, tingling and/or pain.

RECENT STUDY: In two clinical trials, 1,257 people with diabetes took 1,500 milligrams (mg) of ALC, 3,000 mg of ALC or a placebo pill daily for one year. Those who took 3,000 mg of ALC daily experienced a significant reduction in pain.

MY VIEW: While ALC often is prescribed for those with age-related cognitive decline (poor memory) and early-stage Alzheimer's disease, it now should be considered a primary form of treatment for diabetic neuropathy. Take 1,000 mg of ALC three times daily (the same dosing schedule used in the study). ALC has a blood-thinning effect, so check with your doctor before using it if you take a blood thinner, such as *warfarin* (Coumadin).

■

REPORT #22

DIABETES SUPPLEMENTS: WHAT WORKS AND WHAT'S WORTHLESS

Source: **Mark A. Stengler, ND,** naturopathic physician in private practice, La Jolla, CA…associate clinical professor at the National College of Naturopathic Medicine, Portland, OR…author of numerous books, including *The Natural Physician's Healing Therapies* and coauthor of *Prescription for Natural Cures* (both from Bottom Line Books)…and author of the *Bottom Line/Natural Healing* newsletter.

Diabetes and a related condition known as "prediabetes" (a precursor to the full-blown disease) are reaching epidemic proportions in America. I disagree with the commonly held belief that diabetes is mainly caused by genetic factors. Most cases can be blamed on diets that include too much refined sugar, particularly the high-fructose corn syrup that is now used in everything from soft drinks and ice cream to candy and yogurt.

Here, I'll tell you how to effectively control blood sugar (glucose) levels with the right diet and supplements. These strategies have consistently helped many of my patients prevent and treat prediabetes and diabetes.

DIABETIC-FRIENDLY FOODS…

To choose the most healthful foods, many diabetics rely on the glycemic index (GI), a ranking system (on a scale of 0 to 100) that indicates the type of carbohydrate in foods and its potential to raise blood glucose levels. The lower a food's GI, the more beneficial it is for controlling levels of glucose and insulin (a blood-sugar–reducing hormone produced in the pancreas). For example, the GI for cola is 63, while kidney beans have a GI of 23.

Another—and sometimes better—way to analyze the effects of food on your glucose and insulin levels is the glycemic load (GL). While the GI describes the degree to which carbohydrates increase glucose levels (the quality of the carbohydrate), the GL takes into account the quality and the actual amount of carbohydrates found in a food.

As with the GI, the higher the GL, the greater the likelihood that blood glucose and insulin levels will increase. The GL is calculated by multiplying the amount of carbohydrates (in grams) in a specified serving size of food by its GI and then dividing the result by 100.

The GI and GL are not perfect systems. Each of us responds differently to specific foods. However, GI—and, to a greater extent, GL—give us a way to understand how food affects our glucose levels.

MEAL PLANNING...

I encourage patients with diabetes to focus their meal planning on high-fiber foods—in particular, vegetables, legumes, fruit, healthful nuts and seeds, and quality grains. Fiber slows the passage and absorption of food in the intestines, which prevents blood glucose levels from rising rapidly.

I've listed below some foods (and the recommended daily servings) in these categories. You'll also find the GL for each food to show how it can affect your glucose levels. A GL of 20 or more is considered high...11 to 19 is medium...and 10 or less is low. To follow these guidelines, focus on eating foods and meal combinations with GLs that are low and only occasionally medium. If you are obese or your diabetes is not well-controlled, your daily total should be below a GL of 60 (80 or less for a controlled diabetic). This diet helps with weight control, so it is a good eating plan for *everyone*.*

*Since GL is based on multiplying the amount of carbohydrate in a food by its glycemic index, low-carbohydrate foods, such as many types of vegetables and meat, have no GL. To control calories, portion sizes still need to be monitored for meat, dairy and oils.

• *Vegetables.*

GOAL: Five to seven servings daily. A serving is defined as one cup of raw, leafy vegetables...one-half cup of raw, canned or cooked nonleafy vegetables...or three-quarters cup of 100% vegetable juice.

Broccoli (1 cup)..0 GL
Carrots (1 large)..5 GL
Celery (1 cup)..0 GL
Onions (1 medium)...2 GL
Spinach (1 cup) ....0 GL

• *Legumes.*

GOAL: One to two servings daily. A serving is defined as one-half cup of cooked legumes.

Black-eyed peas (½ cup)................................. 13 GL
Kidney beans (½ cup) .... 7 GL
Lentils (½ cup)... 2.5 GL
Peas (½ cup) .... 3 GL
Soy (½ cup of soybeans) .... 1 GL

• *Grains.*

GOAL: Three to five servings daily of unrefined grains. A serving is defined as one slice of bread...one cup of ready-to-eat cereal...or one-half cup of cooked rice, pasta, cereal or oats.

Whole-wheat bread (1 slice) .... 10 GL
Oats (½ cup, cooked) .... 3 GL
Whole-grain cereals (1 cup, Grape-Nuts)......... 15 GL
Brown rice (½ cup, cooked).............................. 6 GL

• *Fruits.*

GOAL: Two to three servings daily. A serving is defined as one medium fruit...one-half cup of raw, canned or cooked fruit...or three-quarters cup of 100% fruit juice.

Apples (1 medium) .... 5 GL
Blueberries (½ cup)... 1 GL
Grapes (½ cup) .... 5 GL
Oranges (1 medium).. 5 GL
Strawberries (½ cup)... 1 GL

• *Protein.*

GOAL: Two to three servings daily. A serving is defined as one or two eggs...or four ounces of meat/poultry.

Eggs (1 large) ....0 GL

Fish, especially cold-water salmon,
    sardines, trout (4 ounces) .... 0 GL
Chicken (4 ounces) .... 0 GL
Turkey (4 ounces)... 0 GL
Beef (4 ounces, lean), two to four times
    a month.. 0 GL
• *Nuts, seeds and oils.*
GOAL: Three to four servings daily. A serving is defined as one-quarter cup of nuts...or one tablespoon of oil.
Almonds (¼ cup).. 0 GL
Cashews (¼ cup)... 1.5 GL
Flaxseeds (2 tablespoons) .... 0 GL
Olive oil (1 tablespoon)....................................... 0 GL
• *Dairy.*
OPTIONAL: One serving daily. A serving is defined as one cup of milk or yogurt...or two ounces of low- or nonfat cheese.
NOTE: Cow's milk is a common allergen.
Cottage cheese (1 cup) .... 0 GL
Cheese (2 ounces) .... 0 GL
For a complete list of the GI and GL of common foods, go to the Web site of the University of Sydney (where the GI and GL were invented) at *www.glycemicindex.com.* Or read *The New Glucose Revolution*, by Jennie Brand-Miller (Marlowe & Company).

SUPPLEMENT ESSENTIALS...

Many different nutritional supplements have been studied for their effects on people with diabetes. Some supplements are especially well-suited, but they can affect the proper dosage of pharmaceutical diabetes medication. Be sure that your blood glucose level is monitored by your doctor and with home testing.

Work with your doctor to introduce one or two supplements (in the order listed below) into your treatment regimen. Gradually add other supplements over a period of weeks or months for optimal nutritional benefit or for help with specific symptoms.

• *Multivitamin/mineral formula.* A high-potency, full-spectrum multivitamin/mineral formula is essential for people with diabetes. Anyone with this disease has a greater need for antioxidants because high glucose levels promote the development of harmful molecules (free radicals) that damage cells. These free radicals create inflammation in cells and accelerate aging. A good multivitamin/mineral formula provides a wide range of antioxidants, including vitamins A, C and E, as well as selenium, *alpha lipoic acid* and many other nutrients.

IMPORTANT: Choose a formula that does not contain iron. Elevated iron levels increase free radical activity.

• *Chromium.* This mineral aids insulin in transporting glucose into cells. Approximately 20 studies have investigated how supplemental chromium affects diabetes. About 60% of diabetes patients who take it report improved glucose control. People with diabetes typically take up to 500 micrograms twice daily. People with kidney disease should not take chromium.

• *Cinnamon.* This popular spice (also available in supplement form) not only tastes good, but also lowers blood sugar levels. In a 2003 study of 60 people with type 2 diabetes, fasting glucose levels were reduced by 18% to 29% after 40 days of taking cinnamon capsules. Those taking a placebo had no significant changes. According to studies conducted at the US Department of Agriculture, cinnamon appears to enhance the activity of insulin. The type of cinnamon used in studies thus far is Cassia cinnamon (*Cinnamomum aromaticum*), which is widely available in the spice section of grocery stores. As a food, use one to one-and-one-half teaspoons daily. I like to sprinkle cinnamon on sliced apples or whole-grain toast. If you prefer a supplement (available at health-food stores), take 1,000 to 2,000 mg daily.

• *Alpha lipoic acid (ALA).* This sulphur-containing, vitamin-like antioxidant has been shown to improve glucose balance for people with type 2 diabetes. A standard daily dose is 300 mg, but up to 1,800 mg daily has been shown to help reduce symptoms of diabetes-related peripheral neuropathy (nerve pain in the extremities), including burning, numbness and/or prickling of the feet and legs. This benefit is most likely due to ALA's potent antioxidant effects. ALA often can improve glucose control and neuropathy pain within four weeks.

• *Coenzyme Q10 (CoQ10).* This supplement prevents and treats high blood pressure in people with diabetes and helps with blood sugar control. This heart-friendly antioxidant also is vital for proper cardiovascular health. I recommend that people with diabetes take 200 to 300 mg of CoQ10 daily.

■

REPORT #23

HIDDEN HEALTH RISKS
THEY DON'T WANT YOU TO KNOW

Sources: **Michael F. Roizen, MD,** chair of the division of anesthesiology, critical care medicine and comprehensive pain management at the Cleveland Clinic... **Mehmet C. Oz, MD,** medical director of the Integrative Medicine Center and director of the Heart Institute at NewYork-Presbyterian Hospital—Columbia University in New York City. Dr. Roizen and Dr. Oz are coauthors of the bestselling *You: The Owner's Manual.* HarperCollins.

Most people unintentionally increase their risk for illness, premature aging and even death simply because they lack key facts about their own bodies.

PROBLEM: Because doctors don't have time to educate patients about everything that could possibly go wrong with their health, you need to have a basic understanding of what kinds of symptoms to watch for...and which medical advice can be trusted.

Some of the most commonly held beliefs are actually the most dangerous...

MYTH: Ulcers aren't contagious. Nearly all ulcers are caused by *Helicobacter pylori* (H. pylori), a spiral-shaped bacterium that penetrates the stomach lining. A blood test can detect H. pylori in people with ulcer symptoms, including pain in the abdominal area just above the navel. Doctors can successfully eradicate H. pylori with a two-week course of antibiotics, but ulcers often return.

REASON: Kissing can transmit the bacterium. Even if an ulcer patient is successfully treated with antibiotics, he/she can reacquire the bacterium—and the ulcer—from H. pylori–infected saliva.

RECOMMENDATION: If you or your spouse or partner has ulcers due to H. pylori, ask your doctor about *both* of you taking antibiotics to avoid reinfecting one another. Also, get a new toothbrush to avoid reinfecting yourself.

MYTH: High blood pressure begins at 140/90. Until recently, doctors didn't consider blood pressure to be elevated unless it was above 140/90. According to the National Heart, Lung, and

Blood Institute, a patient with a reading as low as 120/80 has *prehypertension*—and is at an increased risk for heart disease.

Optimal blood pressure is 115/76. The difference of just a few points might seem insignificant, but patients who maintain blood pressure readings at this level or lower have *half* the cardiovascular risk of those at the higher level of 120/80.

RECOMMENDATION: Because many doctors don't flag blood pressure readings that are only slightly elevated, ask the nurse/technician taking your blood pressure what your reading is. If it is above 115/76, ask your doctor how you can bring it down.

Slight elevations can almost always be controlled with lifestyle changes, such as losing just five to 10 pounds, exercising and increasing fruit and vegetable intake.

MYTH: If your cholesterol levels are normal, you won't have a heart attack. Most heart attack sufferers have normal cholesterol levels. Few people realize that heart attacks are typically caused by blood clots that form on top of irritated, inflamed areas of plaque (a mixture of cholesterol and other substances) on artery walls. When these clots grow, they can lodge in an artery and cause a heart attack.

Lowering LDL ("bad") cholesterol creates a less favorable environment for clot formation. If your doctor says your LDL cholesterol is elevated, it's time to implement lifestyle changes, such as diet and exercise.

Still, some researchers speculate that statins, such as *atorvastatin* (Lipitor), work not so much by lowering cholesterol but rather by reducing the arterial inflammation that promotes clots. In fact, studies have shown that statins reduce heart attack risk even in patients with normal cholesterol levels.

IMPORTANT: Do *not* take more than 100 milligrams (mg) of vitamin C or 100 international units (IU) of vitamin E daily if you are taking a statin. These vitamins inhibit the drug's anti-inflammatory effects.

In addition to statins, there are other effective strategies to help prevent inflammation and clots.

RECOMMENDATION 1: Be sure that you take good care of your teeth. Brush *and* floss daily. Get a professional cleaning twice a year. The bacteria that cause gum disease can also promote inflammation and plaque in the arteries.

RECOMMENDATION 2: Consider aspirin therapy. Ask your doctor about taking two 81-mg "baby" (or half an adult) aspirin daily to reduce arterial inflammation and inhibit clots.

HELPFUL: Buy regular, cheap aspirin. Drink one-half glass of water before and after taking the aspirin. This aids absorption and makes the aspirin less likely to cause gastrointestinal bleeding.

IMPORTANT: Some recent studies have questioned whether aspirin really does help prevent heart disease, but we recommend this therapy for patients who are candidates because it also helps curb the risk for colon, breast, prostate and other types of cancer.

MYTH: Fiber prevents colon cancer. Eating fruits and vegetables can help prevent colon malignancies and other cancers, but research shows that it isn't the fiber in these foods that does the trick—it's the antioxidants.

Although there are many reasons to get plenty of dietary fiber—for example, it prevents constipation, improves digestion and helps lower LDL cholesterol levels—there are other approaches that have been proven to be more effective at preventing colon cancer.

RECOMMENDATION 1: Ask about aspirin. Two baby (or half an adult) aspirin daily reduces your risk of colon cancer by 40%, possibly due to its anti-inflammatory effect. Ask your doctor if aspirin is right for you. It should not be taken with blood thinners.

RECOMMENDATION 2: Boost intake of folate and calcium. People who take at least 400 micrograms (mcg) of folate daily and/or 500 mg of calcium twice daily reduce their colon cancer risk by 30%. The reason for this effect is unknown, but researchers believe these supplements may slow the harmful breakdown of DNA that is associated with cancer.

MYTH: The more you exercise, the better your health. The human body isn't designed to withstand constant stress. People who exercise vigorously for more than about an hour a day don't live longer or healthier lives than those who exercise at moderate levels.

RECOMMENDATION: Get one hour a day of moderate exercise —fast walking, swimming, bicycling, etc. Research shows that this level of activity can make you feel and behave younger.

Regular physical activity promotes weight loss, improves cardiovascular conditioning and bone strength and reduces the risk for diabetes. It's important to remember that exercising for more than one hour doesn't provide additional health benefits but does increase the risk for muscle, bone or joint damage.

MYTH: Diarrhea should run its course. A common misconception is that it's best not to treat diarrhea in order to promote the removal of organisms/toxins that lead to this potentially dangerous condition.

Not true. Untreated diarrhea is more than just uncomfortable. It can remove quarts of water from the body and cause dangerous dehydration within 24 hours, especially in children and older adults.

RECOMMENDATION: Eat chicken soup with rice. The broth and rice provide protective sugars to cells that line the intestine. Drink two quarts of water or juice daily to prevent dehydration. Take readily absorbable, calcium-containing tablets (such as Tums) several times daily. Calcium slows muscular movements in the intestine.

REPORT #24

THE NEXT BIG DRUG SCANDALS

Source: **Jack M. Rosenberg, PharmD, PhD,** director of the International Drug Information Center at the Arnold & Marie Schwartz College of Pharmacy & Health Sciences at Long Island University in Brooklyn, NY.

Over-the-counter (OTC) drugs can be purchased just as easily as a bottle of shampoo or a box of cereal—but that doesn't mean that they're harmless.

Few people realize that in some cases, OTC drugs contain the same amount of an active ingredient as that found in prescription medications. Using OTC drugs incorrectly—for example, taking them for too long or in excessive doses—can cause serious side effects.

EXAMPLE 1: People with arthritis often treat their symptoms with OTC painkillers, such as *ibuprofen* (Advil) or *naproxen*

(Aleve), for months or years—even though the label advises against taking these drugs for more than 10 consecutive days without consulting your doctor. The long-term use of such drugs greatly increases the risk for stomach bleeding as well as heart and/or kidney problems.

EXAMPLE II: If you have hypertension or heart disease, taking a cold remedy that contains *pseudoephedrine*, such as Sudafed, can cause a life-threatening problem such as atrial fibrillation (a heart-rhythm irregularity) or heart attack.

All OTC medications include a standardized "Drug Facts" label (on the outside of the packaging and also in an insert) that details the approved uses of the drug...active ingredients...how to use it...and possible risks. Even though OTC drug labels were simplified in 2002, the information is often confusing and printed in such small type that it's almost impossible to read.

NOTE: The US Food and Drug Administration (FDA) recently has required drug manufacturers to redesign *prescription* drug labels so that they are easier to read.

IMPORTANT: Bring your reading glasses or a small magnifying glass with you and read the OTC drug label *before* leaving the store. If you're purchasing from a drugstore, ask a pharmacist to explain any instructions that you don't understand.

What to look for...

ACTIVE INGREDIENT...

This term refers to the medication that relieves symptoms. There might be dozens of drugs in a pharmacy that have the same active ingredient.

EXAMPLE: Advil Cold & Sinus Liqui-Gels and Motrin Cold & Sinus caplets both contain 200 milligrams (mg) of ibuprofen and 30 mg of pseudoephedrine. Knowing the active ingredient makes it easy to comparison shop for the best price.

WHAT YOU MAY NOT KNOW: Manufacturers occasionally change the active ingredients in OTC products.

EXAMPLE: The antidiarrheal drug Kaopectate once contained a type of clay called *attapulgite*. It was safe for patients who were taking blood-thinning medication. Kaopectate now contains *bismuth subsalicylate*, an aspirin-like ingredient that increases the risk for bleeding in patients taking blood thinners.

INACTIVE INGREDIENTS...

Inactive ingredients are the chemicals that are used as preservatives, binders and colorants/flavors—but have no medical effects.

WHAT YOU MAY NOT KNOW: Some people are allergic to certain inactive (as well as active) ingredients.

EXAMPLE I: Hundreds of products, such as the OTC antihistamine *loratadine* (Alavert) and the OTC pain reliever Arthritis Strength BC Powder, contain the inactive ingredient lactose, a milk sugar that can trigger reactions in patients who are lactose intolerant.

EXAMPLE II: Gluten, a protein found in wheat, barley and rye, should be avoided by people with celiac disease, but starch, maltodextrin and other substances that could contain gluten are common inactive ingredients in both OTC and prescription medications, such as the OTC anti-gas drug Gas-X Regular Strength Chewable Tablets and the fiber supplement Senokot Wheat Bran.

USES...

Known as "indications" on some labels, this term refers to the list of symptoms that a drug is designed to treat.

The FDA allows drug manufacturers to list only uses for which the medication has been proven to be safe and effective.

EXAMPLE: The label on an antihistamine such as *diphenhydramine* (Benadryl) says the drug treats sneezing, runny nose and other allergy symptoms.

WHAT YOU MAY NOT KNOW: It can be risky to take drugs "off-label"—that is, taking a medication for uses other than the indications and/or directions found on the label.

EXAMPLE: Taking high doses of the OTC B vitamin niacin to lower cholesterol is an off-label use. Prescription niacin is approved for lowering cholesterol, but taking it without being monitored by your doctor can lead to liver damage.

WARNINGS...

Many patients ignore the warnings on OTC medications because they assume the drugs must be safe or they wouldn't be sold without a prescription. Not true.

OTC drugs can cause side effects that are just as serious as those caused by prescription drugs. Aspirin and related

drugs, for example, cause more than 100,000 hospitalizations annually in the US.

WHAT YOU MAY NOT KNOW: In addition to explaining the main risks of a medication, "warnings" may include information on who should not take the medication, when to consult your doctor if symptoms persist, when to take medications with foods (or when to avoid certain foods and beverages), whether it's safe to drive, etc.

Even if you've taken a particular OTC drug for years, check the warning label each time you purchase the medication. A drug that was safe when you first started taking it might cause problems if you've begun taking other medications or if the ingredients or your health needs have changed. Always check the expiration date.

FORMS AND FORMULATIONS...

The label on an OTC drug lists the medication's form—tablet, capsule, caplet, etc. The form can affect how quickly the product works...what side effects occur...and how easy it is to take.

Examples...

• *Buffered analgesics (pain relievers)* are made slightly alkaline to protect the stomach. Patients who experience stomach irritation, pain or heartburn from aspirin or similar drugs might do better with a buffered product.

• *Caplets are ordinary tablets* in the shape of a capsule. They're easier to swallow than traditional tablets—an important point for patients who have trouble swallowing. Gelcaps, geltabs and capsules are coated with gelatin, making them also easier to swallow.

• *Timed-release capsules or tablets.* These drugs are designed with various types and layers of coatings around the active ingredients, which allows the medication to be released slowly, resulting in extended drug action.

An enteric-coated drug is treated so that it passes through the stomach unaltered and dissolves in the intestines. Enteric-coated medications take longer to work, so if you have a headache (and do not have a sensitive stomach), it may be better to take regular aspirin than enteric-coated aspirin.

• *Extra-strength drugs* contain a higher dose of the active ingredient. These medications, such as Extra Strength Tylenol, are helpful if the regular dose isn't adequate to control symptoms—and more convenient than taking two or more doses of a lower-dose product.

• *PM (or night formulas)*, including some antihistamines or pain relievers, such as Excedrin PM, can cause drowsiness, so they're meant to be taken at night.

• *Suspension formulas* are liquid medications in which the active ingredient isn't dissolved. They require shaking before use (and typically indicate this on the label).

EXAMPLE: The laxative Phillips Milk of Magnesia is an oral suspension medication.

■

REPORT #25

DEADLY MISTAKES THAT DOCTORS MAKE

Source: **Paul Barach, MD, MPH,** director of the Miami Center for Patient Safety and associate professor of anesthesiology, both at the University of Miami Miller School of Medicine. The Center develops patient-safety courses and guidelines for hospitals and medical schools, researches medical errors at hospitals and teaches the importance of improving communication in clinical settings.

When Dr. Paul Barach was a third-year medical student, an attending physician told him to insert a central intravenous (IV) line into a 75-year-old patient suffering from emphysema. Dr. Barach had never performed the procedure before. Alone and unguided, he wound up puncturing the air sac around the lung, and the patient eventually died of related complications.

Though Dr. Barach went on to an illustrious career, he was haunted by the incident and became driven to understand how medical errors can be prevented. Today, Dr. Barach is one of the country's foremost patient-safety advocates.

We recently spoke with him about the best ways for medical consumers to protect themselves against medical errors.

What are the most common errors?

Medication errors. This includes not only oral medications but also errors involving IV drugs (given through the veins for serious conditions, such as heart attack or stroke) or subcutaneous injections (given beneath the skin, such as a diabetic's insulin shot). The Institute of Medicine estimates that 3% to 5% of all medication is administered incorrectly.

Medication errors include a number of different scenarios and can happen anywhere—in hospitals, doctors' offices and pharmacies. For example, a drug may not be given at exactly the right time, in the right dose or with the right frequency. In most instances, this type of error is minor and has no consequences.

However, IV drugs act much more quickly than oral medications, so those mistakes are frequently irreversible and the consequences are more severe. With chemotherapy, for example, dosing is a very complex process that requires different combinations and amounts of toxic drugs, so there's an even greater risk for harm.

Are certain people at increased risk for medical errors?

Older adults and psychiatric patients all are at high risk. Older adults are more likely to be on multiple medications and less likely to pay close attention when drugs are being administered. Psychiatric patients generally don't ask questions related to medications.

What can patients do to make sure their medication is being administered properly?

Get very clear and very detailed explanations from your provider, beforehand and in writing. Find out what you're going to be taking, for how long and what side effects might occur. Using a polite tone, ask your physician, *Can you please tell me what this drug is for? What are its side effects? What dose should I be on?* Research the medication(s) before you take them. Read about them in a medical reference book at your local library, surf the Internet or talk to your pharmacist. Then make sure you get what you are prescribed. If you have any doubts or questions whatsoever, be sure to speak up.

How can patients protect themselves before they undergo anesthesia?

Patients should insist on meeting their anesthesiologist ahead of time to discuss all of their concerns and to go through their complete medical history. You cannot assume that your anesthesiologist has your records or has reviewed them.

Mention if you or a family member has had trouble with anesthesia or if you have a history of hyperthermia (a rare condition in which the body is susceptible to very high fevers).

Also mention if you have any loose teeth. In rare cases, a patient's teeth are knocked out when the breathing tube is inserted down the throat. Teeth are nicked, chipped or broken in about 500 of 100,000 cases. That's about 0.5% of the time.

A good hospital will always require you to have a preoperative examination with an anesthesiologist. This is the only person who understands how to monitor your medications.

We all know that hospital patients should ask a family member or friend to be on-site to help monitor their care. What should this person be looking for?

Your guardian should know your treatment plan and your medication schedule. He/she should ask your doctor about these facts and write them down. If the doctor has put you on a low-sodium diet, for example, your guardian should ask if the food is low-sodium when it arrives. Your guardian should scrutinize any medicine before it is administered to make sure it's correct. This is especially true if, for example, the patient in the next room has a name that is similar to yours.

What's the best way to choose a care guardian?

Look for someone with common sense, inquisitiveness and assertiveness. Choose a person who will put your interests above everything else and who will be able to stand up for you should a discrepancy arise.

If a health-care provider appears incompetent, should a patient insist on having someone else take over?

That depends. If someone is causing you unusual pain or prodding or poking you too hard during an examination, you should alert the head nurse or attending physician. You even can get up and leave, if necessary.

Sometimes a caregiver can have trouble performing a procedure through no fault of his own. Even the most experienced health-care professional can take 45 minutes to get an IV line into a long-term smoker whose veins are hardened.

If you feel that you are not receiving the caregiver's undivided attention or if there is a lot of noise and confusion in your room, voice your concern.

How common is it for people to die or for serious errors to occur without the patient or family members knowing what went wrong?

No one knows for sure. If you believe that a medical error has occurred, talk to your caregiver. Ask for a full disclosure of

all the facts and a copy of your medical records and charts. If
necessary, you can ask to speak to the head of the department.
If you still are not getting an adequate response or if you feel
you are being stonewalled, contact the head of the hospital.

Documentation has greatly improved over the years, providing more accountability in case of a medical error.

■

REPORT #26

DON'T BECOME A VICTIM
OF MEDICAL NEGLECT

Source: **Pamela F. Gallin, MD,** director and associate professor, pediatric oph-
thalmology, Columbia-Presbyterian Medical Center and Columbia University College of Physicians and Surgeons, both in New York City. She has served on the
White House Health Care Task Force and is author of *How to Survive Your Doctor's
Care.* LifeLine Press.

Even doctors—who know the ins and outs of the health-care
system and get better-than-average care—fall victim to
medical errors and neglect.

EXAMPLE: Four days after I had hand surgery in 1988, I had
incredible pain. The surgeon, thinking I was overreacting,
wouldn't even give me an appointment to see him.

I did get in to see one of his colleagues, who immediately took
off the cast. It had been put on too tightly and was damaging
nerves and impeding circulation. It took six months for the nerves
to recover—and worse, I could have lost the use of the hand.

Time pressures, cost-saving measures and the endless
maze of insurance bureaucracies all guarantee that mistakes
will happen. So now it's up to patients to make sure mistakes
don't happen to them. **HERE'S HOW...**

CHOOSE THE RIGHT HOSPITAL...

Your primary-care doctor is just one of many who will tend
to your care. You want to make sure that *all* of your doctors
and nurses are the best available—and the place to find them
is usually at a major medical center affiliated with a teaching
university.

These hospitals offer the latest and most effective tests and treatments. All of your primary-care doctor's colleagues—such as radiologists, anesthesiologists, etc.—will have similar levels of training. No matter where you live, there's probably a major teaching hospital within a few hours' drive and affiliates even closer to your home.

CAUTION: Many major medical centers lend their names to suburban hospitals and clinics. Don't assume that they all offer the same level of care. If your doctor serves at one of these affiliates, ask if he/she also has privileges at the main institution.

PICK THE RIGHT KIND OF DOCTOR...

Many patients choose family-practice physicians or obstetrician/gynecologists as their primary-care doctors. That's fine if you're young and healthy, but if you have pre-existing conditions or are age 35 or older, your primary-care physician should be an internist.

Internists tend to know more about evaluating—and treating—diseases and are trained to coordinate your overall care if you need multiple doctors. Many internists have additional training in other specialties, such as rheumatology, cardiology or gastroenterology. Pick an internist whose training matches *your* medical needs.

IMPORTANT: Your doctor should be board-certified in his area of expertise. The Web site *www.docboard.org* offers background information on physicians, including notations on disciplinary actions and medical malpractice lawsuits that have been filed.

QUESTION YOUR DIAGNOSIS...

Two equally competent doctors can look at the same test results and arrive at different conclusions.

Always get a second opinion if you've been diagnosed with a serious health problem, such as cancer or a heart condition.

If the second opinion differs from the first, ask doctor No. 2 why doctor No. 1 is mistaken. Get as much information as you can. Don't hesitate to get even a third opinion if the first two are conflicting.

IMPORTANT: Get the second opinion from a doctor who specializes in your condition.

The sister of a friend of mine was told by her internist that her lung cancer had recurred, based on an abnormal chest

X-ray. She got a second opinion from a pulmonary oncologist, who performed several tests, including magnetic resonance imaging (MRI), blood tests and a biopsy. The second doctor determined that the problem was merely inflammation. The internist wasn't a bad doctor. He got it wrong because he wasn't a trained oncologist.

ALWAYS REPEAT "BAD" TESTS...

Diagnostic and treatment errors often are due to faulty tests or an improper interpretation of the results. If a test indicates that you have a serious problem, consider having it repeated. Be especially suspicious when test results that were normal in the past suddenly seem much worse.

IMPORTANT: If your test was done at a small hospital or clinic, have the test results sent to a major medical center for a second opinion. This usually costs $100 to $150, and your insurance may pay for it.

ALSO: Ask that your tests be read by a pathologist or radiologist who specializes in that particular part of the body.

EXAMPLE: If you've had a computed tomography (CT) scan of your head to investigate a possible tumor, the films should be reviewed by a neuroradiologist at a major medical center. A general radiologist who works at a local hospital may misinterpret the findings.

PICK YOUR SURGERY TEAM...

If you need an operation, it's not enough just to choose your surgeon. You also should be involved in picking the anesthesiologist. Anesthesia is one of the most dangerous parts of surgery.

Key points...

• *Ask your surgeon to include an anesthesiologist* who specializes in your condition.

EXAMPLE: A neuroanesthesiologist if you will need to have neurosurgery.

• *Ask for an anesthesiologist who works with your surgeon frequently.* Good teamwork will reduce the risk of complications.

• *Request a board-certified anesthesiologist.* This is especially true if you're having a lengthy or complicated procedure, such as cardiac or abdominal surgery.

■

REPORT #27

DON'T BE DECEIVED BY DRUG COMPANY TACTICS

Source: **Marcia Angell, MD,** former editor in chief, *The New England Journal of Medicine,* and senior lecturer, Harvard Medical School's department of social medicine, Boston. She is a nationally recognized authority in the field of health policy and medical ethics and an outspoken critic of the health-care system. She is author of *The Truth About the Drug Companies.* Random House.

In light of revelations about the harmfulness of the prescription drug *rofecoxib* (Vioxx)—it was taken off the market—and other painkillers, drug companies have come under increased scrutiny.

FACT: Between 1997 and 2001, drug companies tripled the amount of money they spent on direct-to-consumer advertising for prescription drugs—the ads now seen so frequently on television and in newspapers.* The number of retail prescriptions rose from 2.4 billion in 1997 to 3.1 billion in 2001. Those prescriptions carry a total yearly price tag of at least $200 million, with the cost rising about 12% per year, approximately six times the rate of inflation.

But doesn't the increased use of medications signal better health for Americans? Not necessarily.

Marcia Angell, MD, former editor in chief of the prestigious *New England Journal of Medicine,* discussed the claims made by drug companies...

CLAIM: The increased costs of drugs reflect large investments in research and development (R&D).

FACT: Drug companies spend more than twice as much on "marketing and administration" as they do on R&D—31% of sales, compared with 14% in 2003.

Drug industry sources say the R&D cost per drug is $800 million, on average. An independent analysis by the nonprofit consumer advocacy organization Public Citizen shows that the real cost is probably $100 million or less.

Actually, the big drug companies don't develop most of the novel medications. These drugs, such as the cancer medications

*2001 is the most recent year for which information is complete.

paclitaxel (Taxol) and *imatinib* (Gleevec), mostly are the result of taxpayer-funded research at academic institutions or the National Institutes of Health (NIH) or research at small biotechnology companies.

CLAIM: New drugs are constantly being brought to market.

FACT: Of the 487 drugs approved by the US Food and Drug Administration (FDA) from 1998 through 2003, only 32% contained new active ingredients and fewer than half of those (14% of the total) were classified by the FDA as improvements over older drugs.

Most "new" drugs are chemical variations of older drugs already on the market—so-called "me-too" drugs. Companies try to grab a piece of a profitable market by producing a medication similar to a top-selling drug.

EXAMPLE: Mevacor, approved in 1987, was the first cholesterol-lowering statin in the marketplace. Now, there are five more, all variants of the original—Lipitor, Zocor, Pravachol, Lescol and Crestor. Even though Lipitor and Zocor are the top-selling statins, no head-to-head studies have been conducted comparing their effectiveness with *lovastatin* (the cheaper generic form of Mevacor) when taken at equivalent doses.

CLAIM: Scientific studies on drugs are reliable.

FACT: Drug companies have always sponsored almost all research on their drugs, but now they control how the research is done and whether it will be published. Much of this research is seriously flawed, presenting results that cause both doctors and consumers to believe that drugs are a lot better than they are and have fewer side effects than they do. What's more, only favorable results are published. Unfavorable results rarely see the light of day.

CLAIM: Doctors' prescribing habits aren't unduly influenced by drug companies.

FACT: In 2001, the drug industry employed approximately 88,000 sales representatives to visit doctors in their offices and hospitals to promote their products—roughly one representative for every six practicing physicians. Drug reps attend medical conferences and offer doctors expensive gifts. Although some doctors refuse these gifts, many do accept dinners, football tickets, family vacations, etc.

In 2001, drug companies paid more than 60% of the costs for continuing medical education for doctors. Meetings of professional societies, such as the American College of Cardiology and the American College of Physicians, now are largely sponsored by drug companies.

Knowing this, do you think the prescribing habits of doctors in America are based only on the objective evaluations of their patients?

WHAT YOU CAN DO...

To protect yourself against drug industry tactics...

• *Ignore drug ads.* An ad is meant to sell something, not educate or inform. Drug ads are no different. There's a good reason that direct-to-consumer drug ads are illegal in every other developed country (except New Zealand).

• *Be skeptical about new drugs.* When it comes to drugs, newer doesn't necessarily mean better. There are exceptions, but you should make sure your doctor is relying on scientific evidence, not just a sales pitch from a drug company.

• *Watch out for "me-too" drugs.* If a drug is being advertised on TV, it's probably a me-too drug. The drug company is trying to convince doctors and patients—usually in the absence of any scientific evidence—that the "new" drug is better.

• *Always ask for an equivalent generic or over-the-counter (OTC) drug.* Doctors tend to prescribe what the drug company reps who haunt their offices are pushing. There may be a cheaper alternative that's just as effective. Ask about it.

• *Beware of free samples.* Drug reps give doctors free samples of expensive drugs. When the sample runs out, both doctor and patient are in the habit of using that particular drug. If you accept a free sample, be sure there is a compelling medical reason to take that drug.

• *Don't be easily convinced that you have a new disease.* Do you really need to take the me-too antidepressant *paroxetine* (Paxil) for "social anxiety disorder"—when you thought you were just shy?

• *Give your doctor permission not to prescribe.* Many doctors assume—correctly, in many cases—that a patient won't feel satisfied unless he/she leaves the office with a prescription.

TELL YOUR MD: *If I don't need a prescription drug, then don't prescribe one.*

■

REPORT #28

WARNING: READ THIS BEFORE HAVING OUTPATIENT SURGERY

Source: **Charles B. Inlander,** health-care consultant and president of the non-profit People's Medical Society, a consumer health advocacy group in Allentown, PA. He is author of many books on consumer health issues, including *Take This Book to the Hospital with You.* St. Martin's.

Few things in medicine have changed more radically in the past 20 years than the location where people go for surgery. More than 1,500 different surgical procedures that previously were performed only on an inpatient basis, including the removal of cataracts and colon polyps, now can be performed on outpatients who enter a facility in the morning and leave later the same day. Although outpatient surgeries are cheaper and often safer (largely because of significantly lower infection rates), a successful outcome typically depends on the type of outpatient facility you choose for your procedure.

Key points to consider…

• *Doctors' offices.* You are not paying the high overhead associated with a hospital or free-standing surgical center, so procedures performed in a doctor's office can cost up to 50% less than those in the other settings—but they come with greater risk. That's because doctors' offices are not accredited by any private or government oversight agency. In fact, under current state laws, any licensed doctor (physicians must be licensed by the state in which they practice) can perform just about any surgical procedure in his/her own office without any special approval. Because of this, insurance companies and Medicare may not pay for a procedure performed in a physician's office. Check to see if your insurer will pay for the procedure you need with the doctor you are considering. If not, ask the company for a list of doctors' offices approved for payment.

• *Free-standing surgical centers.* Often called "surgi-centers," these usually are a better choice than a doctor's office. These facilities, often independently owned by physicians or entrepreneurs, tend to be better regulated. Most states require them to be licensed, usually by the state health department. That means they are inspected and must meet certain standards for safety, infection control and other quality-related factors. They also can be accredited by the Accreditation Association for Ambulatory Healthcare or the Joint Commission on the Accreditation of Healthcare Organizations. Although accreditation is voluntary for surgi-centers, it's smart to choose a facility that is accredited by one of these organizations.

• *Hospital-owned outpatient facility.* This usually is your best choice for outpatient surgery. Since it is a part of a hospital, it must meet the same regulatory standards and accreditation requirements as the rest of the hospital (even if it is not located at the hospital site). These standards and requirements are much more strict and comprehensive than for other settings. Unlike a doctor's office or a surgi-center, hospital-owned outpatient facilities collect important data, such as infection rates. Many hospitals now are making that information publicly available. Ask for the annual surgical and outpatient report. If it's not available, consider another facility.

■

REPORT #29

BE SURE YOUR SURGEON KNOWS WHERE TO CUT

Source: **Richard Croteau, MD,** executive director for patient safety initiatives, Joint Commission on Accreditation of Healthcare Organizations, Oakbrook Terrace, IL.

Incision sites must now be marked by surgeons. The US rules, established by the Joint Commission on Accreditation of Healthcare Organizations, also require the surgical team to take a "time-out" before starting surgery. This ensures that the right patient is on the table and that all doctors, nurses and other medical personnel agree on what procedure is to be performed. Mistakes, such as operating on the wrong side of a patient or performing the wrong procedure, were reported about 300 times from 1995 to 2004.

IF YOU'RE UNDERGOING SURGERY: Ask your surgeon to mark the surgical site when you are awake. Otherwise, ask a friend or family member to observe.

■

REPORT #30

UNEXPECTED SOURCES OF LETHAL INFECTIONS

Source: **Charles B. Inlander,** health-care consultant and president of the non-profit People's Medical Society, a consumer health advocacy group in Allentown, PA. He is author of many books on consumer health issues, including *Take This Book to the Hospital with You.* St. Martin's.

Some people may be aware of the dangers of deadly infections acquired in hospitals. According to the Centers for Disease Control and Prevention (CDC), these infections kill approximately 100,000 patients each year, seriously harm almost 2 million additional people and add more than $5 billion to annual health-care costs. The CDC also estimates that up to half of these infections are preventable, if only hospital personnel would take infection control more seriously—primarily by washing their hands.

However, hospitals aren't the only place where unsuspecting medical consumers can acquire deadly infections. You also can get an infection at outpatient surgical and emergency centers, nursing homes, assisted-living facilities—even in your doctor's office. Not a single state routinely inspects nonhospital medical facilities for infection-control practices, nor do states require these facilities to report infections that might have been caused by treatments received there. That means it's up to you—the patient—to take steps that will lower your risk for infection. **BEST STRATEGIES...**

• *Look for clean hands.* You may have heard it before, but you cannot afford to ignore this advice. In fact, the CDC reports that staff not washing their hands is the number-one reason that infections spread. Don't let anyone—not even a doctor or a nurse—touch you unless he/she has washed his hands in your presence. If a health-care worker comes into the examining room with gloves on, ask him to remove those gloves, wash his hands and put on new gloves. It's been found that, in rare cases, personnel wear the same gloves all day long!

• *Insist on clean equipment.* For example, make sure a doctor or nurse wipes the flat surface (diaphragm) of his stethoscope with alcohol before listening to your chest. Studies show that stethoscopes can be contaminated with *staphylococcus aureus* and other deadly bacteria that can easily spread if the equipment is not cleaned.

• *Beware of urinary catheters.* Infections caused by urinary catheters are a problem, especially in nursing homes and assisted-living facilities. The longer the catheters stay in, the greater the risk for infection. Too often, catheters are inserted in patients for the convenience of the staff, simply because they do not have the time (or desire) to bring a bedpan or change a diaper. Unless there is a medical reason for a urinary catheter, insist on a bedpan or diaper. It can save your life—or that of a loved one.

• *Ask about presurgical antibiotics.* When it comes to infection, outpatient surgery is just as risky as inpatient surgery. Research now shows that many patients should be given an antibiotic within one hour of surgery. Unfortunately, busy health-care workers often forget to administer it. So when your surgery is scheduled, talk to your doctor about receiving a presurgical antibiotic. If it is recommended, ask about the antibiotic as soon as you arrive at the facility or doctor's office.

REPORT #31

MIGRAINES GONE IN AN HOUR!

Source: Headache.

The US Food and Drug Administration (FDA) has approved the intraoral vasoconstriction (IVC) device for treating migraines. Migraine patients often have an inflamed area above the upper molar teeth. Chilling the area reduces pressure on the maxillary nerve and relieves migraine pain in less than one hour in 80% of patients.

REPORT #32

"NANO-GEL" MAKES YOU PAIN-FREE FOR WEEKS

Source: **Mark A. Stengler, ND,** naturopathic physician in private practice, La Jol-la, CA...associate clinical professor at the National College of Naturopathic Medi-cine, Portland, OR...author of numerous books, including *The Natural Physician's Healing Therapies* and coauthor of *Prescription for Natural Cures* (both from Bottom Line Books)...and author of the *Bottom Line/Natural Healing* newsletter.

Not long ago, a 60-year-old woman came to my office suf-fering from severe arthritis pain in both hands. I gave her a bean-sized dab of a homeopathic gel that she applied directly to the skin on her hands. After a few applications in the span of 30 minutes, her pain was reduced by 90%. She did not need to apply the gel again for two weeks.

I witnessed a similar result with a retired National Football League player. He had severe chronic hip pain from past inju-ries. With one application of the gel, his pain was relieved by 70% for two full days.

The relief that these people experienced has given them each a new lease on life. *But here's the best news*—unlike pharmaceutical pain relievers, which often cause gastrointes-tinal upset or damage to internal organs, natural therapies can reduce pain without adverse effects.

WHAT ARE YOU TAKING FOR PAIN?...

Most Americans take too many pharmaceutical pain re-lievers. An estimated 175 million American adults take over-the-counter (OTC) pain relievers regularly. About one-fifth of Americans in their 60s take at least one painkiller for chronic pain on a regular basis.

There has been a lot of news about the life-threatening risks of anti-inflammatory medications such as *rofecoxib* (Vioxx) and *celecoxib* (Celebrex), two pain relievers that had been heavily prescribed by conventional doctors to treat the chronic pain of arthritis and similar conditions. Vioxx was pulled off the market by its manufacturer, Merck, following research that linked it to increased risk of heart attack and stroke. Celebrex is undergoing post-marketing clinical trials to determine whether it poses similar risks and now carries warnings about adverse effects, such as abdominal pain, diarrhea and edema (water retention).

Of course, pain-relieving drugs can be a blessing in the event of injury, severe acute migraines or diseases, such as terminal cancer. A number of years ago, when I had a wisdom tooth extracted, I received a local anesthetic. Afterward, I went to an acupuncturist for pain relief so I wouldn't need any painkillers. For about one hour after the acupuncture, I was fine—but then the pain-relieving endorphins wore off. I tried a few natural remedies, but when the pain became excruciating, I resorted to the OTC pain reliever *acetaminophen* (Tylenol). That did the trick.

But many people use painkillers on a regular basis for several months or even years, which increases the risk of dangerous side effects. For instance, people who rely on acetaminophen increase their risk of developing stomach ulcers, liver disease and kidney disease. If you regularly take Celebrex or an OTC nonsteroidal anti-inflammatory drug (NSAID), such as aspirin or *naproxen* (Aleve), you run the risk of kidney and stomach damage. Regular use of NSAIDs also increases the risk of heart attack, according to the US Food and Drug Administration (FDA).

BETTER RESULTS, FEWER RISKS...

Before you take any remedy, it's important for your doctor to identify what is causing your pain. Remember, pain is your body's distress signal that something is being irritated or damaged. Sometimes we protect ourselves by reacting instinctively. If you touch something hot, for example, you eliminate the pain by quickly pulling back your hand.

But what if your back hurts? You may need a pain reliever —but back pain also can be a signal that you're harming your body by bending or sitting the wrong way. You may need to address the underlying cause to prevent further injury. Pain receptors are found in the skin, around bones and joints— even in the walls of arteries. If a muscle is torn, for example, a pain signal is released from fibers in the shredded tissue.

In light of the dangers from prescription and OTC drugs, what safe alternatives are available to you? There are many natural supplements that I recommend.

NATURE'S PAIN RELIEVERS...

If you take prescription or OTC pain medication, work with a naturopathic physician, holistic medical doctor or chiropractor who will incorporate natural pain fighters into your treatment regimen. With his/her help, you may be able to reduce your dosage of pain medication (natural pain relievers can be used safely with prescription or OTC painkillers)—or even eliminate the drugs altogether.

Natural pain-fighting supplements are even more effective when combined with physical therapies, such as acupuncture, chiropractic, magnet therapy or osteopathic manipulation (a technique in which an osteopathic physician uses his hands to move a patient's muscles and joints with stretching, gentle pressure and resistance). Physiotherapy (treatment that uses physical agents, such as exercise and massage, to develop, maintain and restore movement and functional ability) is also helpful.

Here are—in no special order—the best natural pain relievers, which can be taken alone or in combination...

• *White willow bark extract* is great for headaches, arthritis, muscle aches and fever. In Europe, doctors prescribe this herbal remedy for back pain, and recent research supports this use. One study conducted in Haifa, Israel, involved 191 patients with chronic low-back pain who took one or two doses of willow bark extract or a placebo daily for four weeks. Researchers found that 39% of patients taking the higher dose of willow bark extract had complete pain relief, compared with only 6% of those taking a placebo. The participants who benefited the most took willow bark extract that contained 240 milligrams (mg) of the compound *salicin*, the active constituent in this herbal remedy. (Aspirin is made from *acetylsalicylic acid*, which has many of the chemical properties of salicin. However, aspirin can cause gastrointestinal ulceration and other side effects, including kidney damage.) Willow bark extract is believed to work by inhibiting naturally occurring enzymes that cause inflammation and pain.

I recommend taking willow bark extract containing 240 mg of salicin daily. In rare cases, willow bark extract can cause mild stomach upset. Don't take willow bark if you have a history of ulcers, gastritis or kidney disease. It should also not be taken by anyone who is allergic to aspirin. As with aspirin, willow bark extract should never be given to children under age 12 who have a fever—in rare instances, it can cause a fatal disease called Reye's syndrome. Willow bark extract has blood-thinning properties, so avoid it if you take a blood thinner, such as *warfarin* (Coumadin). For low-back pain, you may need to take willow bark extract for a week or more before you get results.

• *Methylsulfonylmethane (MSM)* is a popular nutritional supplement that relieves muscle and joint pain. According to Stanley Jacob, MD, a professor at Oregon Health & Science University who has conducted much of the original research on MSM, this supplement reduces inflammation by improving blood flow. Your cells have receptors that send out pain signals when they're deprived of blood. That's why increased blood flow diminishes pain.

MSM, a natural compound found in green vegetables, fruits and grains, reduces muscle spasms and softens painful scar tissue from previous injuries. A double-blind study of 50 people with osteoarthritis of the knee found that MSM helps relieve arthritis pain.

Start with a daily dose of 3,000 to 5,000 mg of MSM. If your pain and/or inflammation doesn't improve within five days, increase the dose up to 8,000 mg daily, taken in several doses throughout the day. If you develop digestive upset or loose stools, reduce the dosage. If you prefer, you can apply MSM cream (per the label instructions) to your skin at the painful area. This product is available at health-food stores and works well for localized pain. MSM has a mild blood-thinning effect, so check with your doctor if you take a blood thinner.

• *S-adenosylmethionine (SAMe)* is a natural compound found in the body. The supplement is an effective treatment for people who have osteoarthritis accompanied by cartilage degeneration. SAMe's ability to reduce pain, stiffness and swelling is similar to that of NSAIDs such as ibuprofen and naproxen, and the anti-inflammatory medication Celebrex. There's also evidence that SAMe stimulates cartilage repair, which helps prevent bones from rubbing against one another. A 16-week study conducted at the University of California, Irvine, compared two groups of people who were being treated for knee pain caused by osteoarthritis. Some took 1,200 mg of SAMe daily, while others took 200 mg of Celebrex. It took longer for people to get relief from SAMe, but by the second month, SAMe proved to be just as effective as Celebrex.

Most patients with osteoarthritis and fibromyalgia (a disorder characterized by widespread pain in muscles, tendons and ligaments) who take SAMe notice improvement within four to eight weeks. Many studies use 1,200 mg of SAMe daily in divided doses. In my experience, taking 400 mg twice daily works well. It's a good idea to take a multivitamin or 50-mg B-complex supplement daily while you're taking SAMe. The vitamin B-12 and folic acid contained in either supplement help your body metabolize SAMe, which means that the remedy goes to work faster.

• *Kaprex* is effective for mild pain caused by injury or osteoarthritis. It is a blend of hops, rosemary extract and *oleanic acid*, which is derived from olive leaf extract. Rather than blocking the body's pain-causing enzymes, these natural substances inhibit pain-causing chemicals called *prostaglandins*.

In a study sponsored by the Institute for Functional Medicine, the research arm of the supplement manufacturer Metagenics, taking Kaprex for six weeks reduced minor pain by as much as 72%. I recommend taking one 440-mg tablet three times daily. Kaprex is manufactured by Metagenics (800-692-9400, *www. metagenics.com*), the institute's product branch. The product is sold only in doctors' offices. To find a practitioner in your area who sells Kaprex, call the toll-free number. Kaprex has no known side effects and does not interact with other medications.

• *Proteolytic enzymes,* including *bromelain, trypsin, chymotrypsin, pancreatin, papain* and a range of protein-digesting enzymes derived from the fermentation of fungus, reduce pain and inflammation by improving blood flow. You can find these natural pain fighters at health-food stores in products labeled "proteolytic enzymes." Take as directed on the label. Bromelain, a favorite of athletes, is available on its own. Extracted from pineapple stems, bromelain reduces swelling by breaking down blood clots that can form as a result of trauma and impede circulation. It works well for bruises, sprains and surgical recovery. If you use bromelain, take 500 mg three times daily between meals.

Repair is a high-potency formula of proteolytic enzymes that I often recommend. It is manufactured by Enzymedica. (To find a retailer, call 888-918-1118 or go to *www.enzymedica.com*.)

Take two capsules two to three times daily between meals. Don't take Repair or any proteolytic enzyme formula if you have an active ulcer or gastritis. Any enzyme product can have a mild blood-thinning effect, so check with your doctor if you take a blood thinner.

• *Pain Med* is the homeopathic gel that gave such quick relief to the patients I described at the beginning of this article. It is remarkably effective for relieving the pain of arthritis, muscle soreness and spasms, sprains, strains, stiffness, headaches (especially due to tension) as well as injuries, including bruises.

Pain Med is a combination of nine highly diluted plant and flower materials, including *arnica*, *bryonia*, *hypericum* and *ledum*. Like other homeopathic remedies, it promotes the body's ability to heal itself. A bean-sized dab works well for anyone who has pain. It should be spread on the skin around the affected area. Following an injury, use it every 15 minutes, for a total of up to four applications. As the pain starts to diminish, apply less often. Do not reapply the gel once the pain is gone. Pain Med does not sting, burn or irritate the skin. It is clear, has no odor, does not stain and dries quickly. Because it has so many uses and works so rapidly, Pain Med is a good first-aid remedy to have on hand. To order, contact the manufacturer, GM International at 800-228-9850.

REPORT #33

A SMARTER WAY TO TREAT CHRONIC PAIN

Source: **Mark Allen Young, MD,** licensed acupuncturist and chairman of physical medicine and rehabilitation, Maryland Rehabilitation Center, Baltimore. He is author of *Women and Pain.* Hyperion. *www.womenandpain.com.*

If you rely exclusively on aspirin, ibuprofen or another over-the-counter (OTC) medication to control pain, you may be shortchanging yourself.

Few people realize it, but there is often a much more effective way to combat pain. A comprehensive treatment approach, including strategic eating habits, supplements, exercise and medication, stops pain for a variety of common ailments.

The following strategies* may be effective for you...

ARTHRITIS...

OTC pain-relieving remedies used alone are woefully inadequate for osteoarthritis pain. **BETTER APPROACHES...**

• *Eat avocados and soy foods,* such as tofu and tempeh. They reduce inflammation and pain, while promoting cartilage growth. Consume these foods daily.

• *Eat more fish.* The fatty acids in cold-water fish (such as salmon, mackerel and tuna) will help prevent body chemicals called prostaglandins from triggering inflammation. Consume at least three servings weekly.

• *Perform cardiovascular exercise daily.* Swimming and brisk walking are ideal. Both reduce pressure on joints by strengthening surrounding muscles. Vigorous exercise also triggers the release of endorphins, the body's natural painkillers.

• *Take glucosamine.* This supplement nourishes cartilage and gives it more elasticity. Some studies show that glucosamine temporarily relieves pain as well as ibuprofen, and it is unlikely to cause side effects.

TYPICAL DOSAGE: 500 milligrams (mg) three times daily.

BACK PAIN...

Half of all adult Americans suffer from back pain. More than 90% of these cases involve a muscle spasm that is caused by injury, poor posture or excessive body weight.

If you are experiencing back pain that is accompanied by pain or numbness in the buttocks, legs or feet, see a doctor immediately. These can be symptoms of a more serious condition, such as disk or nerve damage. **BUT WHEN PAIN IS THE ONLY SYMPTOM...**

• *Apply a pain-relieving ointment twice daily.* The active ingredient in these products temporarily prevents pain signals from reaching the brain.

GOOD CHOICES: ArthroMax, Bengay and Joint-Ritis.

• *Learn to relax.* Stress accentuates your perception of pain... promotes muscle tightness...and increases the risk for injury.

*Before trying these approaches, consult your doctor to determine the cause of your pain.

Devote at least 40 minutes daily to meditation, exercise, yoga or another relaxing activity.

• *Stretch and strengthen abdominal and back muscles.* Four times per day, lie on your back with knees slightly bent... tighten muscles in the belly and buttocks...and push the lower back against the floor.

Hold for five seconds, then relax and repeat.

FIBROMYALGIA...

This misunderstood and frequently misdiagnosed condition is characterized by widespread, chronic pain involving multiple "tender points" in the upper neck, back, shoulders and hips.

Conventional treatments—painkillers, antidepressants, muscle relaxants and injections of anesthetics—are rarely effective.

ADDITIONAL OPTIONS...

• *Consume apples and/or apple juice.* They contain *malic acid,* a substance that appears to ease fibromyalgia pain. Consume at least two apples or two eight-ounce glasses of juice daily.

• *Try acupuncture.* It triggers a massive release of endorphins, which can reduce pain for more than a week after each treatment.

To locate an acupuncturist in your area, contact the American Academy of Medical Acupuncture at 323-937-5514, *www.medi calacupuncture.org.*

• *Do not give up on exercise.* People with fibromyalgia often stop exercising because it's painful. But inactivity weakens muscles and makes them more sensitive to pain. Low-impact aerobic conditioning exercises, such as swimming, stationary bicycling or stretching, are often helpful.

HEADACHE...

The vast majority of headaches are tension headaches, caused by a muscle spasm in the head or neck. OTC pain-relievers provide temporary relief. ALSO IMPORTANT...

• *Drink more water.* Dehydration is a leading cause of headaches. Consume at least eight eight-ounce glasses of water every day.

• *Avoid caffeine.* It increases muscle tension. Drink no more than one cup of coffee per day.

• *Practice acupressure.* It minimizes pain and stiffness.

WHAT TO DO: Firmly press your finger or thumb into the hollow between the skull and the back of the neck. Hold for 90 seconds. Repeat three times daily.

• *Take feverfew.* This herb contains *parthenolide*, an agent that reduces spasms in blood vessels in the head. Feverfew works for migraines as well as tension headaches.

MUSCLE STRAIN...

This usually involves damage to ligaments, the cords of fibrous tissue that bind bones together. **TO REDUCE PAIN AND SPEED HEALING...**

• *Take a hot bath.* Warmth relieves muscle spasm.

• *Apply ice within 24 hours of the injury...*wrap it with an elastic bandage...and elevate it above heart-level to reduce swelling.

• *Take vitamin E.* It blocks the effects of harmful molecules (free radicals) that result from muscle injuries.

• *Apply capsaicin cream.* Capsaicin is the potent compound that makes chili peppers hot. The OTC ointment warms the area and reduces pain. Apply twice daily.

GOOD CHOICES: Zostrix and Cap-Max Plus.

REPORT #34

STOP PAIN FAST WITH SELF-HYPNOSIS

Source: **Bruce N. Eimer, PhD,** clinical psychologist and hypnotherapist in private practice, Philadelphia. He is author of *Hypnotize Yourself Out of Pain Now! A Powerful, User-Friendly Program for Anyone Searching for Immediate Pain Relief.* New Harbinger.

As a clinical psychologist, I have specialized for 18 years in treating people with chronic pain. But only after a car accident left me in severe, unrelenting pain did I come to fully appreciate the power of hypnosis to pick up where drugs, physical therapy and surgery leave off.

WHY HYPNOSIS?...

Hypnosis is an altered state of consciousness. It magnifies your ability to focus and temporarily sharpens your concentration.

All hypnosis is *self*-hypnosis. Even if the state is achieved with the help of an expert, you can become hypnotized only if you allow yourself to be.*

The nature of hypnosis makes it helpful for chronic pain. It is a state of concentrated attention, which in itself can reduce pain and emotional anguish associated with physical suffering. It also eases tension and curbs insomnia.

ENTERING THE HYPNOTIC STATE...

The first step in hypnosis is called *induction*. In this process, you employ techniques that focus your attention (on the ticking of a metronome or the sound of a voice, for example) and provide suggestions to deepen relaxation.

Try this two-minute induction method, which many people find effective...

Raise one hand. Concentrate on a single finger, with your eyes open (staring at the finger) or closed (imagining it). Let the other fingers fade away from your awareness.

As you continue to concentrate, feel your hand and arm start to grow heavier. Lower your arm slowly, and allow yourself to enter into a comfortable state of relaxation.

By the time your hand comes all the way down and is resting in your lap or on the armrest of your chair, your eyes should be closed and you should feel relaxed. Focus on your breathing. Feel your belly expand with each inhalation and contract as you exhale.

To relax more deeply, close your eyes and imagine you are walking down a set of 20 stairs. Feel the thick, plush carpeting beneath your feet...the smooth, polished wood of the handrail.

With each step, you fall into a deeper state of relaxation. At the bottom of the stairs, you find a door. Open it, and "enter" the place where you feel most happy, content and pleased (a balmy beach, a cool mountain meadow or a sidewalk café in Paris). Imagine this "favorite place" in detail, and stay there as long as you want.

*To locate a qualified clinical hypnosis practitioner in your area, contact the American Society of Clinical Hypnosis at 630-980-4740, *www.asch.net.*

To emerge from the hypnotic state, walk back up the stairs, feeling more awake with each step. When you reach the top, you'll feel alert and refreshed.

The more often you repeat the induction, the better you will get at it. Practice at least twice a day, for 10 minutes each time.

USING THE HYPNOTIC STATE...

After you have practiced induction daily for three weeks, you should be able to elicit deep relaxation at will and enter your "favorite place" whenever you need a stress break or a respite from pain.

Once you've mastered induction, the following techniques should be added. Practice the technique of your choice for 10 minutes daily.

• *Distraction.* Most people naturally cope with pain by focusing their attention elsewhere. For a simple distraction technique, rub the fingers of one hand together. Concentrate on the sensations in your fingers, the texture of the skin and the temperature.

Do this *before* inducing the hypnotic state. This will give your subconscious the suggestion that you can distract yourself the same way whenever you feel discomfort. After the first month, you'll find that even when you are in your normal waking state, you'll be able to divert your attention away from pain more effectively.

• *Dissociation.* This is perhaps the most powerful way to cope with severe pain. Your pain is not gone, but your subconscious mind takes over the task of feeling the pain while your conscious mind is relaxed.

Practice dissociation by visualizing your shadow. It moves with you and is attached to your body, but it is not inside your body. While in a hypnotic state, imagine your shadow...then visualize yourself merging with it.

Put the pain in your shadow. Then imagine yourself floating away from the shadow and the pain. The pain is in your shadow, but not in your body.

• *Self-suggestion.* This technique helps develop attitudes and beliefs that strengthen your ability to cope with pain.

Choose messages that have particular meaning for you, and write them in a journal or on index cards. Repeat one to yourself three times before inducing the hypnotic state.

Some helpful self-suggestions...
• *I am in charge.*
• *I can manage the pain. I can stand this.*
• *Whenever I feel stressed, I accept the feelings and stay calm.*
• *I take satisfaction every day in handling my problems better and better.*

■

REPORT #35

TRY THE MIND–BODY CURE

Source: **John E. Sarno, MD,** professor of clinical rehabilitation medicine at New York University School of Medicine, and an attending physician at the Rusk Institute of Rehabilitation Medicine, both in New York City. He is author of *The Mindbody Prescription.* Warner Books.

From backaches and headaches to wrist pain caused by carpal tunnel syndrome, chronic pain continues to be an enormous problem in this country. Why is that? Because the average doctor persists in the mistaken belief that pain is a structural disorder.

In my opinion, most chronic pain is the result of an *emotionally induced* physical condition—which, in turn, is the result of hidden conflict between our conscious and unconscious minds.

This mind–body cycle of pain is known as *tension myositis syndrome* (TMS).

THREE-STEP SEQUENCE...

Chronic pain typically occurs as a result of a three-step sequence...

1. *You're under pressure.* It might be psychological stress caused by perfectionism or another self-induced pressure...or an external pressure, such as a demanding boss.

2. *Growing pressure gives rise to rage and frustration.* These feelings lie within the *unconscious* mind only. That's because they're simply too frightening to be acceptable to your conscious mind.

You're not even aware of their existence—despite the fact that they can be *very* intense.

3. To keep angry feelings from spilling over into consciousness, your subconscious mind directs your attention to your body. It does so by activating your autonomic nervous system, which controls digestion, respiration, circulation and other involuntary functions.

Upon activation, the autonomic nervous system reduces blood flow to a particular muscle, tendon or nerve. Exactly which part of the body is affected varies. The decrease in circulation deprives the tissues of oxygen. That causes pain.

STOPPING CHRONIC PAIN...

To stop pain caused by TMS, you *don't* need painkilling medication...or surgery...or physical therapy. What you need is an *understanding* of the three-step sequence.

Once you acknowledge that pain stems from the subconscious mind's efforts to protect your conscious mind from troubling emotions, you can get on with the cure...

• *Have a doctor rule out physical causes.* You must be absolutely certain that there is no serious disease causing your pain—cancer, for example.

IMPORTANT: Despite what many doctors believe, spinal disc abnormalities are rarely the cause of back pain.

In one study, back pain sufferers proved to be no more likely to have spinal disc degeneration or bone spurs than people who did not have back pain.

In a similar study, researchers detected disc abnormalities in 64 people—*none* of whom had back pain.

• *"Talk" to your brain.* This sounds silly, but it works. If you feel a twinge of pain, silently tell your brain that you *know* what it is doing—you can even tell it to increase the blood flow to the painful area.

Put your brain on notice that you're no longer going to let yourself be affected by its efforts to shield you from any negative emotions.

• *Accept that pain is caused by repressed emotions.* It can be very hard to admit that emotions are causing your pain—especially if a doctor has told you that the culprit is a slipped disc or another structural problem...or physical stress, such as that caused by typing for hours a day.

Of course, your conscious mind is desperately trying to deny that emotions are the cause. It doesn't want to experience those emotions—or even admit that they exist.

• *Make a written list of the possible sources of your psychological stress.* In making the list, remember that most distress is internally generated. **TWO COMMON EXAMPLES...**

EXAMPLE I: Perfectionism. Because you're so eager to excel at everything you do, you're highly critical of yourself—and overly sensitive to criticism from others.

EXAMPLE II: The need to be liked. You try to be *good* and *nice* to everyone—because you want everyone's love, admiration and respect. "Goodism" is just as stressful as perfectionism—and just as likely to cause frustration and rage.

External causes of distress might include a mean boss, an argumentative spouse, a meddlesome relative or another person with whom you have a difficult relationship.

It could also be serious financial trouble or simply a sense of having too little time to get things done.

Even happy experiences—marriage, job promotion, a new baby—create pressure. And pressure creates unconscious rage.

By reading and rereading your list—and reminding yourself of the true cause of your pain—you'll "cure" the pain.

Most people who use this technique become pain-free within eight weeks.

• *Review your list on a daily basis.* Spend at least 30 minutes a day thinking about each item on your list and how it could be causing pressure in your life.

Resolve to take action to defuse the pressures you can...and to accept the pressures you cannot change.

• *Visualize your rage.* Imagine yourself in a blind fury. That is the experience your unconscious mind is having to cope with on a continuing basis.

Now consider what might happen if you gave free rein to your rage. You could ruin your marriage, lose your job—even wind up in jail.

Your conscious mind is as frightened of these experiences as you are. That's why it chooses to hide your rage from you.

• *Resume physical activity.* Once your pain has largely subsided, go back to exercising, lifting heavy objects, using a computer keyboard, etc.

Start slowly, and build up over a period of weeks.

If you're afraid to resume normal activity, it means that your unconscious mind is still in charge. You've got more mind–body work to do.

• *Understand "location substitution."* Say you've just gotten over a bad case of back pain—and now your elbow has started to hurt.

Chances are that the brain has simply picked a *new* spot in your body to cause pain to distract you from your rage.

Realize the same pain process is happening once again— only in another part of your body. Once again, the pain should disappear.

STAY PAIN-FREE FOREVER...

To keep pain at bay, you must continually remind yourself that pressure causes unconscious, frightening rage...and your brain distracts your attention from that rage by creating pain.

Tell yourself this again and again, and you should stay pain-free for the rest of your life.

■

REPORT #36

THIS 10-STEP PROGRAM TREATS PAIN VERY, VERY EFFECTIVELY

Source: **Dharma Singh Khalsa, MD,** founding director of the Acupuncture, Stress Medicine and Chronic Pain Program, University of Arizona College of Medicine, Phoenix.

Twenty-five million Americans are bedeviled by some form of chronic pain—sciatica, migraine, arthritis, muscle pain, etc. There are effective ways to curb chronic pain, but these *aren't* the ways typically recommended by mainstream physicians.

In addition to surgery and narcotics, mainstream doctors often recommend nonsteroidal anti-inflammatory drugs (NSAIDs) like *ibuprofen* (Motrin) to their patients with chronic pain.

These drugs can be highly effective against acute pain, such as sprains or toothaches. But they're less effective against chronic pain. And—NSAIDs sometimes cause bleeding ulcers and other side effects.

Here are 10 pain-relieving strategies that really work...

• *Eat more fish and poultry.* Doctors often prescribe *fluoxetine* (Prozac) for chronic pain. This prescription antidepressant helps curb pain by boosting levels of the neurotransmitter *serotonin* in the brain. Serotonin blocks synthesis of *substance P*, one of the main chemical messengers involved in chronic pain.

But many people can keep serotonin levels high simply by eating foods rich in *tryptophan*, an amino acid that the body converts into serotonin.

Two excellent sources of tryptophan are poultry and fish. If you have chronic pain, try eating three ounces of either one five days a week.

In addition to blocking substance P, serotonin helps make people less aware of pain by improving mood and regulating disturbed sleep cycles.

• *Eat a banana every day.* Most chronic pain stems from arthritis, muscle pain or another inflammatory condition, which invariably goes hand in hand with muscle spasms. These spasms contribute to chronic pain.

Eat one banana a day—along with a bit of the lining of the peel that you've scraped off with a spoon. Doing so will supply you with lots of magnesium and potassium. Both minerals help control spasms.

• *Get regular exercise.* Exercise triggers the synthesis of natural painkillers known as *endorphins*.

If you're experiencing severe pain, of course, you probably don't feel like doing vigorous exercise. That's fine. Endorphin synthesis can be triggered by any form of activity that pushes the body a bit harder than it's accustomed to.

If you've been sedentary for a long time, something as simple as rotating your arms for a few seconds can work. So can sitting in a chair and raising your legs a few times.

• *Take steps to control psychological stress.* Stress plays a central role in chronic pain. Meditation and other relaxation techniques reduce muscle spasms, limit the release of pain-causing stress hormones and improve breathing. Each of these helps reduce pain intensity.

One recent study found that pain sufferers who meditated for 10 to 20 minutes a day visited a pain clinic 36% less often than did their nonmeditating peers.

WHAT TO DO: Carve out at least 15 minutes of quiet time each day. If you aren't comfortable meditating, use the time to pray...visualize a tranquil scene...or sit quietly.

• *Avoid harmful fats.* Red meat and cooking oil stimulate the production of *arachidonic acid*, a compound that the body converts into hormone-like substances that trigger inflammation. These substances are known as *prostaglandins*.

Chronic pain sufferers should avoid red meat entirely...and use cooking oil sparingly.

• *Take omega-3 fatty acid supplements.* Taking 1,000 to 3,000 milligrams (mg) of fish oil or flaxseed oil each day helps block the synthesis of prostaglandins.

In addition to blocking prostaglandin synthesis, a type of omega-3 fatty acid known as *eicosapentaenoic acid* (EPA) improves circulation by making the platelets—cell-like structures that are responsible for blood clotting—less "sticky." This helps keep blood from pooling and causing inflammation and irritation.

Fatty acid supplements are unnecessary for individuals who eat cold-water, dark-flesh fish several times a week. Salmon, tuna, mackerel and sardines all fit the bill.

• *Take a vitamin B complex supplement.* Chronic pain is often accompanied by fatigue. When you feel more energetic, your pain is more manageable.

Ask your doctor about taking a daily supplement that contains at least 50 mg of B complex vitamins.

Vitamin B helps increase energy levels by facilitating the production of ATP, the high-energy compound found in mitochondria, the "power plants" inside cells.

• *Season food with turmeric.* Its primary constituent, *curcumin*, has been shown to be as effective at relieving pain as cortisone or ibuprofen—without any risk for side effects. A pinch or two a day is all you need.

• *Try acupuncture.* There's now solid evidence that acupuncture can be more effective than drug therapy for relieving many types of chronic pain.

Acupuncture that is done by a physician seems to be especially effective. So-called medical acupuncture often involves the application of electrical current to needles inserted into the skin. This variant of traditional acupuncture is called electroacupuncture.

For referral to an acupuncturist in your area, contact the American Academy of Medical Acupuncture at 323-937-5514, *www.medicalacupuncture.org.*

• *See a chiropractor or osteopath.* Most physicians rely upon drug therapy and surgery for controlling pain. Chiropractors and osteopaths incorporate physical manipulation into their treatments. For back pain especially, manipulation often works better than drugs or surgery.

■

REPORT #37

"SANDY'S CURE" FOR CHRONIC ARTHRITIS

Source: **Mark A. Stengler, ND,** naturopathic physician in private practice, La Jolla, CA...associate clinical professor at the National College of Naturopathic Medicine, Portland, OR...author of numerous books, including *The Natural Physician's Healing Therapies* and coauthor of *Prescription for Natural Cures* (both from Bottom Line Books)...and author of the *Bottom Line/Natural Healing* newsletter.

Sandy had been suffering from rheumatoid arthritis for 16 years. This inflammatory disease is characterized by joint pain on both sides of the body, most often in the hands, wrists and knees. It is an autoimmune condition—that is, the body's immune system attacks its own tissue, causing the cartilage in the joints to degrade over time. Sandy, a 43-year-old homemaker, had constant pain and inflammation in her hands and wrists.

When I first saw her, she was taking two prescription anti-inflammatory medications—*methotrexate* (Rheumatrex), which also is used as a chemotherapy agent, and *hydroxychloroquine* (Plaquenil). To make matters worse, she had been in a car accident a year before, which injured her hands and back, further aggravating her condition. In addition to her pain, Sandy's digestion was not good—she was prone to diarrhea, gas and bloating—and for the past five years, she had not slept well.

Understandably, Sandy was concerned about the potential toxicity of her medications. For example, methotrexate can cause liver damage and anemia.

Sandy and I discussed the potential triggers of rheumatoid arthritis—stress (which was high in her life), food sensitivities, hormone imbalances, poor digestion, environmental toxins and nutritional deficiencies.

I started Sandy on enzymes that aid digestion, fish oil, a proteolytic enzyme (to reduce inflammation) and a formula containing the hormone *melatonin* and the amino acid *5-hydroxytryptophan* to help her sleep. I had her tested for hormone imbalances as well as food and environmental sensitivities. I also tested the absorption status of her small intestine.

The tests showed that she had a mild problem with malabsorption—the food she ate was not being broken down and absorbed properly. This validated my prescription for supplements that support digestion. Hormone testing showed that her thyroid was underactive, so I prescribed natural thyroid hormone. The allergist I work with found that Sandy had several food sensitivities—to wheat, tuna, onions, yams and other foods. I suggested that she rotate these foods, since it is difficult to avoid them indefinitely. To reduce the reactions triggered by her overactive immune system, I also recommended that she take desensitization drops, with a homeopathic dilution of the foods to which she was sensitive.

On her follow-up visit two months later, Sandy reported that she no longer had any symptoms of arthritis in her joints and had stopped her medications (with her rheumatologist's knowledge). She did experience a mild flare-up midway through her menstrual cycle, indicating a hormone connection. For this, I prescribed the homeopathic remedy Pulsatilla, known for its hormone-balancing properties. Now, a year later, Sandy experiences only minor, occasional arthritis flare-ups and has been able to reduce the number of supplements she uses.

■

REPORT #38

BEDSORE RELIEF

Source: **Mark A. Stengler, ND,** naturopathic physician in private practice, La Jol-la, CA...associate clinical professor at the National College of Naturopathic Medi-cine, Portland, OR...author of numerous books, including *The Natural Physician's Healing Therapies* and coauthor of *Prescription for Natural Cures* (both from Bottom Line Books)...and author of the *Bottom Line/Natural Healing* newsletter.

If you have never had a bedsore, you might not realize how serious they can be. They affect up to 10% of hospitalized patients and develop when the blood supply to the skin is cut off by pressure and/or friction between skin and bed sheets or a gown. Perspiration, which irritates skin, makes infection more likely. Prevention techniques include frequent turning and repositioning (with help from hospital staff, if needed), adding padding to beds and wheelchairs, and keeping skin clean and dry. Unfortunately, once bedsores develop, they are often slow to heal.

A recent study published in *Clinical Nutrition* involved 16 hospitalized patients, ages 37 to 92, who were divided into three groups. All participants ate the same food. One group received nothing additional. The second group was given two high-protein/energy supplements per day. The third group was given protein/energy supplements containing extra vita-min C (500 mg), zinc (30 mg) and L-arginine (9 grams).

RESULT: Patients receiving the basic high-protein supple-ment showed no better bedsore healing than those receiving no supplements—but those receiving the additional vitamin C, zinc and L-arginine healed significantly faster.

MY TAKE: L-arginine is involved in tissue repair and im-mune function support. It is found in dairy, meat, poultry, fish, nuts and chocolate—but during times of stress, the body cannot produce enough to meet increased requirements. Vi-tamin C and zinc also are known to support immune function and tissue repair. People who are bedridden or susceptible to bedsores should take supplements of vitamin C, zinc and L-arginine at the doses used in this study. If you have kidney disease, check with your doctor first.

REPORT #39

DO YOU SUFFER FROM CHRONIC NECK PAIN?

Source: **Robert Swezey, MD,** clinical professor of medicine at the University of California at Los Angeles, School of Medicine, and founder of the Santa Monica, CA–based Swezey Institute.

Seven out of 10 Americans experience neck pain at some point in their lives. Fifteen percent suffer from chronic neck pain.

GOOD NEWS: Whether it's caused by long hours of computer work or driving, arthritis, age-related disk damage or muscle spasms, neck pain can almost always be prevented. **HERE'S HOW...**

• *Never sleep on your stomach if you already have neck pain.* When sleeping on your back or side, use a neck (cervical) pillow to keep your neck and head in a comfortable position.

Cervical pillows—soft in the middle and firm on the sides—are available at orthopedic-supply stores for about $30.

ALTERNATIVE: Fold an ordinary pillow once lengthwise and fasten around the middle with a necktie or sash.

• *Maintain good posture.* When driving, talking on the phone or doing any other activity that stresses your neck, perform the following *1-2-3-2 posture check* as often as you need to remind yourself of good posture.

1. *Place your right index finger next to your right eye.* Focus on an object in front of you at eye level.

2. *Place your index and middle fingers of your right hand on your chin,* keeping your eyes level. Pull your chin inward until you feel a gentle stretch at the back of your neck, keeping your eyes level.

3. *Place the tips of your middle three fingers of your left hand*

on the top of your head. Push your head up against your fingertips and feel your entire spine lengthen as your head assumes its proper position. Repeat step 2.

• *Design a comfortable work space.* When working at a desk, use a padded, adjustable chair with movable arms to support your forearms and allow your shoulders to relax. Keep your feet flat on the floor—or on an adjustable footstool with your knees slightly higher than your hips.

If you're using a computer, position the monitor just below eye level. Place all documents so that you can read them without turning your head.

• *Strengthen your neck.* **PERFORMED DAILY, THIS ISOMETRIC EXERCISE STRENGTHENS THE NECK MUSCLES...**

• Sit comfortably with your chin level. Place the palm of your right hand against your forehead. Support your elbow with your left hand.
• Exhale slowly while pushing your forehead into your palm and resisting with your hand. Hold for three seconds. Repeat two times.

FOR PAIN RELIEF...

For mild to moderate pain, over-the-counter nonsteroidal anti-inflammatory drugs (NSAIDs), such as *ibuprofen* (Advil) or *naproxen* (Naprosyn), are the first choice. **ALSO HELPFUL...**

• *Cold compresses.* Most neck pain will be relieved if you apply a cold pack for 20 minutes. Or use a flexible package of frozen vegetables. If necessary, repeat once every hour.

TO AVOID FROSTBITE: Wrap the cold pack in a thin towel.

• *Soft cervical collar.* Sold in orthopedic-supply stores for about $30, this device is designed to support your neck in a comfortable position. The collar should allow your head to tilt slightly downward so that your chin can rest on the front of the collar. Until pain subsides, wear it when doing any activity that stresses your neck.

Simple exercises performed three to four times per day or as often as needed can also help relieve the muscle tension that fuels neck pain. If you are wearing a cervical collar, take it off before doing these exercises.

For mild to moderate pain, try this gentle stretch...

• *Intermediate neck rotation.* Sit comfortably with your chin level. Slowly roll your head downward, lowering your chin onto your chest. Let your head hang, feeling a stretch in the

back of your neck. Keep your chin close to your chest, and rotate your head to the right, feeling a stretch on the left side of your neck. Hold for six seconds, then bring your head back to center position and rotate to the left. Repeat three times.

For severe pain, perform the following exercise, which increases motion to the muscles connecting the neck and shoulders...

• *Shoulder shrug with a downward stretch.* Sit comfortably with your chin level. Lift your shoulders up toward your ears until you feel your upper shoulder muscles tighten. Hold for six seconds. Let your shoulders gently fall and reach toward the floor until you feel a stretch in your neck and upper back. Hold for six seconds. Repeat three times.

WHEN TO SEE A DOCTOR...

If self-treatment and exercise do not relieve severe neck pain within two days—or one week if pain is mild to moderate—see a doctor.

An orthopedist, neurosurgeon or physiatrist (a physician who specializes in rehabilitation medicine) is your best option. Make sure the physician you choose has expertise in neck disorders.

The doctor will probably order an X ray and perhaps a magnetic resonance imaging (MRI) scan or computed tomography (CT) scan. Treatment may include a firm cervical brace, ultrasound, massage and/or prescription medications.

For severe pain, your doctor may prescribe a narcotic painkiller, such as *hydrocodone* (Vicodin) or *propoxyphene* (Darvon). If necessary, the painkiller can be supplemented with a muscle relaxant, such as *cyclobenzaprine* (Flexeril) or *carisoprodol* (Soma), and/or a prescription-strength NSAID. If this doesn't help within one week, the next step is cortisone injections.

Regardless of your underlying problem, surgery has potential risks and should be considered only *after* conservative treatments have failed.

CAUTION: In rare cases, neck pain can indicate a fracture, spinal cord injury, tumor, slipped disk or infection. SEE A DOCTOR IMMEDIATELY IF YOU EXPERIENCE...

• *Neck pain accompanied by fever, chills and weight loss.*

• *Severe headache or dizziness.*

• *Numbness, tingling or weakness of the arms and/or legs.*

- *Incontinence of the bowel or bladder.*
- *Intolerable pain.*
- *Pain that has no obvious cause or is accompanied by swelling not due to a muscle spasm.*

Illustrations by Shawn Banner.

■

REPORT #40

NATURAL RELIEF FOR CROHN'S DISEASE AND IBS

Source: **Tim Koch, MD,** chief, section of gastroenterology, West Virginia University School of Medicine, Morgantown.

Peppermint oil relieves the painful cramping brought on by Crohn's disease and *irritable bowel syndrome* (IBS).

HELPFUL: Place one drop of the oil in a cup of warm water, add some sugar, if desired, and drink the mixture 15 to 30 minutes before eating—or when symptoms begin.

WARNING: Don't take peppermint oil without water, and stop taking the mixture if it causes heartburn. Peppermint oil can be purchased at most health food stores.

■

REPORT #41

THE SPEED CURE FOR IBS

Source: **Mark A. Stengler, ND,** naturopathic physician in private practice, La Jolla, CA...associate clinical professor at the National College of Naturopathic Medicine, Portland, OR...author of numerous books, including *The Natural Physician's Healing Therapies* and coauthor of *Prescription for Natural Cures* (both from Bottom Line Books)...and author of the *Bottom Line/Natural Healing* newsletter.

Probiotics are the beneficial bacteria (or "flora") that are found throughout the digestive and urinary tracts. They are a normal part of the immune system and help your body fend off infection, synthesize certain vitamins and absorb nutrients. People with immune or digestive problems (like Irritable Bowel Syndrome [IBS]), and those who have recently been on antibiotics, should take probiotics. Common examples of probiotics are *Lactobacillus acidophilus* and *Bifidobacterium lactis*.

However-*, quality can be a big problem with probiotics. An independent analysis by ConsumerLab.com of 25 different probiotic products found that eight "contained less than 1% of the claimed number of live bacteria or of the expected minimum of one billion."

I have found that most patients respond better to products containing five billion or more active organisms as a daily dose. People with diarrhea and extreme bloating often respond better to starting doses of 30 billion to 50 billion organisms per day for a month, then switching to five billion. I tell patients to take probiotics for two months or until symptoms are gone. (Acute diarrhea should improve within two days.)

Probiotics are best taken 30 minutes after meals or between meals so that there is less chance that the good bacteria will be destroyed by stomach acid. Some products in pill and capsule form are enteric-coated to avoid this problem. High-quality brands available at health-food stores include DDS-Multi Flora ABF by UAS Laboratories (800-422-3371, *www.uaslabs.com*) and Bio-K+ by Bio-K+ International (800-593-2465 or to find a retailer, go to *www.biokplus.com*).

■

REPORT #42

NATURAL WAY TO TREAT CONSTIPATION

Source: **Victor S. Sierpina, MD,** associate professor of family medicine, University of Texas Medical Branch, Galveston.

Corn syrup, long used as a folk remedy, will draw water into the bowels to soften stools, making them easier to pass.

RECIPE: Drink one tablespoon of corn syrup stirred into a glass of warm water twice a day for one or two days.

CAUTION: Don't use this remedy if you're diabetic, dehydrated or taking diuretic medication, such as *furosemide* (Lasix) or *triamterene* (Dyrenium) and *hydrochlorothiazide* (Maxzide).

■

REPORT #43

QUICK HERBAL RELIEF FOR INDIGESTION

Source: **Chanchal Cabrera,** herbalist in private practice, Vancouver, BC, and member, American Herbalists Guild, Cheshire, CT.

Rosemary is often effective in treating indigestion, gas and bloating.

FOR BEST RESULTS: Take as a tea or tincture 15 minutes *before* eating. That helps maximize the effect of the herb's bitter compounds, which promotes the flow of digestive juices.

TO PREPARE THE TEA: Add one teaspoon of dried rosemary to one cup of boiling water. Steep for 10 minutes, then strain. Or, add 10 to 20 drops of tincture to one cup of water.

■

REPORT #44

HOW TO CURE STOMACH AILMENTS NATURALLY

Source: **Rob Pyke, MD, PhD,** Ridgefield, CT–based internist and clinical pharmacologist. He is author of *Dr. Pyke's Natural Way to Complete Stomach Relief—Great Foods and Holistic Methods to Cure Your Upper Digestive Tract Forever.* Prentice Hall.

Whether it's heartburn, an ulcer or acid reflux disease, stomach distress is so common that many of us simply learn to live with it. Either that, or we take an over-the-counter (OTC) remedy and hope for the best. Only 10% of people who suffer from stomach problems consult a doctor.

As an internist and clinical pharmacologist, I'm well-versed in the conventional treatment of all gastrointestinal conditions. Prescription drugs are the primary defense. Some doctors may also counsel their patients to reduce stress, exercise regularly and lose weight to ease stomach problems.

But in 1994, my views on gastrointestinal ailments changed drastically—when I became the patient.

I was suffering from gastritis, an inflammation of the stomach lining. I also had heartburn and *gastroesophageal reflux disease* (GERD). That is a condition that results whenever the contents of the stomach "backwash" into the esophagus and cause irritation.

The gastroenterologist I consulted prescribed the medication *omeprazole* (Prilosec). But two weeks later, my condition still had not improved.

A review of the gastrointestinal tract showed hundreds of little holes in my stomach. That was the last straw. I decided to stop being a "passive patient," relying only on what my doctor told me. I researched conventional and alternative treatments and created a self-healing program that addresses the causes—not the symptoms—of stomach problems.

CAUTION: Before beginning self-treatment, consult a physician about your stomach problem. THIS IS ESPECIALLY TRUE IF YOU ARE EXPERIENCING SYMPTOMS SUCH AS...

• *Stomach pain that lasts more than one hour twice a week.*

• *Loss of appetite or unwanted weight loss.*

• *Blood in your stool* or a darkening of the stool's color.

• *Vomiting episodes that produce "coffee grounds" (dark matter that contains blood).*

• *Difficulty swallowing.*

• *Pain that occurs when using nonsteroidal anti-inflammatory drugs (NSAIDs) or while drinking alcohol or eating spicy foods.*

SELF-CARE STRATEGIES...

In addition to following your physician's advice, here's how to increase your chances of getting relief from stomach problems...

• *Avoid all offending foods.* Most people know the worst stomach offenders—hot peppers, peppermint, chocolate, soda, onions and nuts. But there are less obvious triggers, such as butter, milk, ice cream, coffee and tea. These offenders add or promote stomach acid or open the valve from the stomach to the esophagus, which can result in reflux.

• *Eat the right foods.* Artichokes (try out canned artichoke hearts in salad) and sauerkraut nourish friendly digestive-tract bacteria. Low-fat soy milk and yogurt buffer stomach acid. Papaya and pineapple contain helpful digestive enzymes.

• *Eat six small meals each day instead of three large ones.* You'll produce less stomach acid. Reducing meal size also helps to prevent reflux, the "burp up" sensation that occurs when food and stomach acid back up into the esophagus.

• *Drink no more than one cup of a beverage during each meal.* The more you drink, the more likely your food is to back up into the esophagus. Fluids also dilute digestive enzymes, which convert food into molecules that can be easily absorbed by the intestine.

IMPORTANT: Drink at least eight eight-ounce glasses of water daily. Be sure to drink them between your meals. This helps dilute residual stomach acid.

• *Take 15 minutes or longer to eat each meal.* Most of us don't chew our food well enough. This means that large pieces of food enter the stomach, which can promote indigestion and cause the stomach to empty slowly. This results in excess acid and more opportunity for reflux to develop. Thoroughly chewing your food leads to better digestion.

• *Watch your body position.* To prevent indigestion and reflux, stay upright for at least two hours after eating.

To help stomach patients avoid nighttime reflux, many doctors suggest placing wooden blocks under the feet at the head of the bed. This can work—but if you move around, you run the risk of knocking the bed off the blocks.

BETTER WAY: Get a five- or six-foot wedge of foam from a medical-supply store. The foam should be four inches thick at the head and gradually taper down. Wrap it in a small mattress cover.

BONUS: The wedge enables you to adjust only your side of the bed without disturbing your partner.

• *Ask your doctor about using vitamin supplements and herbs.* Taking certain vitamins and herbs helps prevent and treat stomach conditions.

To decrease stomach acid, consider taking 400 international units (IU) of vitamin E daily. Vitamin C (250 milligrams daily in buffered or ester form) helps heal stomach ulcers.

IMPORTANT: Ask your doctor about taking these in addition to a regular multivitamin, especially because taking more than 200 IU of vitamin E may be dangerous.

Deglycyrrhizinated licorice, aloe vera and chamomile with catnip can also ease stomach upset. These are available at health food stores as capsules, gels, liquids or tea bags. Follow label instructions.

■

REPORT #45

ANTI-DIARRHEA ROOT

Source: **Annemarie Colbin,** certified health education specialist and founder, Natural Gourmet Cookery School, New York City. She is author of several books, including *Food and Our Bones: The Natural Way to Prevent Osteoporosis.* Plume.

Most Southerners are only too familiar with kudzu. This hardy vine—which was imported from Japan a century ago to control soil erosion—has flourished in the South's warm climate, spreading relentlessly over gardens, lawns and houses.

It turns out that the root of this pesky plant has medicinal value. Cooked into a thick broth, it soothes and relaxes the gastrointestinal tract, providing relief from indigestion, heartburn and diarrhea.

Kudzu can also help relieve psychological stress. There's even some evidence that it relieves cravings for alcohol.

Unlike conventional drugs, kudzu provides relief without causing unpleasant side effects. Over-the-counter diarrhea remedies, for example, sometimes lead to constipation.

Kudzu starch is sold in health food stores as *kuzu*—its Japanese name. Pure kuzu is a lumpy white powder. If it's sold as a fine powder, it may be adulterated.

It generally costs $4 to $5 for 3½ ounces.

TO PREPARE KUDZU BROTH: Mix one tablespoon kuzu with one cup cold water until completely dissolved.

Cook on medium heat, stirring continuously. The mixture will thicken and then turn clear upon boiling.

Remove from heat, then add natural soy sauce (shoyu or tamari) to taste—about one tablespoon. Shoyu and tamari are available at health food stores and some supermarkets.

Eat up to one cup of kuzu broth a day until symptoms ease.

IMPORTANT: If discomfort is severe—or lasts more than two days—consult your doctor.

■

REPORT #46

NATURAL TREATMENT FOR INDIGESTION

Source: **Rosario Cuomo, MD,** assistant professor, clinical and experimental medicine, University of Naples "Federico II," Naples, Italy.

More than 60% of people who drank a glass of carbonated water daily experienced a reduction in bloating, nausea, belching, pain and other symptoms of indigestion and constipation, according to a two-week study.

THEORY: Carbonated water will stimulate the proximal (or upper part) of the stomach, which promotes more efficient digestion. Carbonated water may also increase the efficiency of gallbladder emptying.

IF YOU SUFFER FROM INDIGESTION AND CONSTIPATION: Ask your doctor if drinking carbonated water—in addition to other treatment strategies, such as a high-fiber diet—may be beneficial.

■

REPORT #47

COVERED-UP CAUSES OF FOOD POISONING

Source: ABCnews.com.

A 12-year-old middle-school student got national attention when her science project revealed that the ice in some fast-food restaurants harbored more *E. coli* bacteria than toilet water from the same restaurants.

THEORY: Ice machines are rarely cleaned and people use unwashed hands to scoop the ice.

■

REPORT #48

OILS THAT IMPROVE HEALTH

Source: **Victoria Edwards,** founder, Aromatherapy Institute & Research, Fair Oaks, CA, quoted in *Self*, 4 Times Square, New York City 10036.

Eucalyptus is an antibacterial that soothes acne and relieves sinus congestion.

Geranium soaks up facial oiliness and can also tighten skin temporarily.

Lavender soothes tension headaches and migraines.

Rose hydrates and soothes sensitive, dry, itchy or inflamed skin.

Tea tree fights athlete's foot, dandruff, insect bites, cold sores and acne.

CAUTION: Except for lavender and tea tree, don't apply full-strength oils directly to skin. Dilute in a vegetable carrier oil such as almond oil or grape seed oil.

■

REPORT #49

SAVE YOUR EYESIGHT, NOW

Source: Studies quoted in *Health*, 2100 Lakeshore Dr., Birmingham, AL 35209.

People who eat at least five servings of vegetables a week cut their risk in half of suffering *macular degeneration*—the most common cause of blindness in older Americans. Researchers believe that antioxidants in vegetables tie up oxygen molecules known as "free radicals," which otherwise damage the eyes over time. Also, the vitamin A in vegetables prevents loss of night vision.

■

REPORT #50

DR. COFFEE, MD

Source: **Tomas de Paulis, PhD,** coffee chemist and research assistant professor of psychiatry, Institute for Coffee Studies, Vanderbilt University Medical Center, Nashville.

The health benefits from drinking coffee continue to be reported—and to the extent where they almost seem too good to actually be true.

Coffee decreases diabetes risk. Drinking six cups a day slashed risk of diabetes by 54% for men and 30% for women in an 18-year Harvard study. Even drinking only one cup a day was found to reduce risk by several percent.

At least six additional studies indicate coffee drinkers reduce their risk of Parkinson's disease by up to 80%.

And other studies have reported that drinking at least two cups of coffee a day can reduce risk of colon cancer by 25%, risk of gallstones by 50% and risk of liver cirrhosis by 80%.

There's even evidence that coffee drinking offsets some of the health damage caused by smoking and excessive drinking—those who engage in such health vices but also drink coffee have been reported to suffer less heart and liver damage than those who don't.

And other studies have indicated coffee may help to control asthma, relieve headaches, lift spirits and even prevent cavities.

Coffee can also increase athletic performance and endurance—until recently, it was a controlled substance at the Olympic Games.

Moreover, coffee is even good for children. One study in Brazil indicated that children (average age, 12) who drank coffee with milk were less prone to depression and were more alert in school. No study indicates that coffee consumed in reasonable amounts is in any way harmful for children.

■

REPORT #51

FLATTEN YOUR BELLY FOR LIFE

Source: **Chih-Hsing Wu, MD,** associate professor at the Obesity Research Center, department of family medicine, National Cheng Kung University Medical College, Tainan, Taiwan, and the leader of a study of more than 1,100 people, reported in *Obesity Research.*

A recent study of more than 1,100 people found that those who drank tea at least once a week for more than 10 years had 20% less total body fat and 2% less abdominal fat than those who drank none. The study took into account life-style factors, including age, physical activity and food intake. Results applied to black, green and oolong tea.

THEORY: Tea may increase metabolic rate while lowering absorption of sugars and fat-producing molecules.

■

REPORT #52

THE ASTONISHING 60-MINUTE DEPRESSION CURE

Source: **Mark A. Stengler, ND,** naturopathic physician in private practice, La Jolla, CA...associate clinical professor at the National College of Naturopathic Medicine, Portland, OR...author of numerous books, including *The Natural Physician's Healing Therapies* and coauthor of *Prescription for Natural Cures* (both from Bottom Line Books)...and author of the *Bottom Line/Natural Healing* newsletter.

Isn't it strange when some wholesome-looking actor appears on a TV commercial to promote a pharmaceutical? The ad tells you how great the drug is, then proceeds with a long, rapid-fire list of potential side effects. What a contradiction!

It's hard to believe, but Americans spend close to $200 billion each year on prescription drugs. Now, many people are concerned about the side effects of these medications—and with good reason. Each year, 2.9% to 3.7% of hospitalizations in the US are due to adverse reactions to medications.

The solution is to get healthy—and stay healthy—using natural methods. Many nutritional supplements can be used safely and effectively in place of prescription medications. Whether you're treating depression, heartburn, high blood pressure, elevated cholesterol or any number of other common ailments, there are excellent natural alternatives.

CAUTION: Do *not* stop taking a prescription drug or begin using a supplement unless you are being monitored by a health professional.

Natural alternatives work best when combined with diet and lifestyle improvements, particularly regular exercise, stress-reduction techniques and adequate sleep.

Sertaline (Zoloft), *escitalopram* (Lexapro) and *fluoxetine* (Prozac) are the most popular prescription antidepressants sold in the US. They belong to a class of drugs called selective serotonin reuptake inhibitors (SSRIs). *Serotonin*, a neurotransmitter (chemical messenger) produced by nerve cells in the brain, plays an important role in balancing mood. SSRIs temporarily block serotonin from returning to the neuron that released it, boosting the amount of available serotonin.

Potential side effects of SSRIs include drowsiness, nervousness, insomnia, dizziness, nausea, tremors, loss of appetite, headache, diarrhea, dry mouth, irregular heartbeat, skin rash, weight loss or weight gain, and activation of mania in patients with bipolar disorder (also known as manic-depressive illness). These drugs also can cause sexual side effects, including loss of libido and decrease in the intensity of orgasms. In July 2005, the FDA warned that children and adults taking antidepressants should be monitored for signs of worsening depression or suicidal thoughts.

NATURAL ALTERNATIVES: Try them in this order for six to eight weeks. If effective, continue indefinitely. You can take more than one at a time.

• *S-adenosylmethionine (SAMe)*, a nutritional supplement derived from the amino acid *methionine*, is excellent for mild to moderate depression. SAMe is thought to work by increasing the production of mood-boosting neurotransmitters. Some studies that have been conducted have shown SAMe to be as effective as pharmaceutical antidepressants—or, in some cases, even more so. Take 400 milligrams (mg) two or three times daily on an empty stomach. Do not use this supplement if you are taking an antidepressant or antianxiety medication—or if you have bipolar disorder. Like SSRIs, SAMe may activate a manic phase in bipolar patients.

• *5-hydroxytryptophan (5-HTP)* is a quick-acting, mood-enhancing amino acid that can work in as little as 60 minutes. I recommend it for my patients with mild to moderate depression. In the body, 5-HTP is converted into serotonin, helping to raise levels of this mood-balancing neurotransmitter. Take 100 mg two to three times daily on an empty stomach. Do not take 5-HTP in combination with pharmaceutical antidepressant or antianxiety medication.

• *St. John's wort* is an herb that is widely used in Europe to treat depression. In a review of 23 studies, it was found to be as effective as pharmaceutical therapy for mild to moderate depression. I recommend taking 600 mg of a 0.3% hypericin extract in the morning and 300 mg in the afternoon or evening. St. John's wort should not be used by women who take birth control pills or by anyone taking HIV medication or immune-suppressing drugs. Do not take St. John's wort with antidepressant or antianxiety medication.

• *Fish oil* has been shown to help mild to moderate depression. Take a formula that contains 1,000 mg of combined *docosahexaenoic acid* (DHA) and *eicosapentaenoic acid* (EPA) daily. Nordic Naturals and Carlson's both make good formulas that are available at health-food stores. Fish oil can be taken for an indefinite period of time.

• *B vitamins* improve the efficiency of many functions, including the conversion of glucose to fuel and the synthesis of neurotransmitters. Deficiencies of B vitamins (notably B-3) can lead to anxiety and agitation. Take a 50-mg B complex daily for as long as you like.

■

REPORT #53

COVERED-UP FOOD CURES FOR ANXIETY

Source: **Carolyn Chambers Clark, EdD,** board-certified advanced nurse practitioner, mental health specialist and faculty member in the health services doctoral program at Walden University, Minneapolis. She is the author of *Living Well with Anxiety: What Your Doctor Doesn't Tell You...That You Need to Know.* Collins.

Anxiety is a normal reaction to the stresses of everyday living. For example, everyone feels insecure or worried at times. It's also common to feel anxious about job interviews, public speaking and meeting new people. But approximately 40 million American adults experience anxiety that is so persistent or excessive at some point during their lives that it interferes with their ability to function.

Anxiety disorders are among the most common mental health problems in men and women. Health effects associated with anxiety include high blood pressure, tension headache, diarrhea and fatigue.

When people suffering persistent anxiety seek help, doctors typically prescribe anti-anxiety drugs, such as *alprazolam* (Xanax).

WHAT MANY PEOPLE DON'T REALIZE: Drugs used to treat anxiety can be addictive and create severe withdrawal symptoms when patients try to stop using them. They also may be harmful to the kidneys and liver.

ARE YOU AT RISK?...

Anxiety is first learned by being around anxious parents or caregivers. If you have an excitable personality, which may be your temperament or genetic-based, you are more prone to anxiety.

Abuse victims and people who witness death, such as hospital workers, soldiers and firefighters, are especially prone to anxiety.

As a holistic nurse practitioner who has grappled personally with anxiety at different times during my lifetime, I've spent more than 30 years devising an effective nondrug approach to help myself and the people I treat. **BEST STRATEGIES...**

REVIEW YOUR DIET...

• *Caffeine* triggers the release of the brain chemical *norepinephrine*, which increases alertness. However, caffeine also causes your body to release adrenaline—just as if you're undergoing stress.

It's best to forgo caffeine altogether. Slowly withdraw over a few days. Try adding more decaffeinated coffee to your cup and less caffeinated coffee. Remember that coffee isn't the only source of caffeine. Tea, cola, cocoa and many over-the-counter medications, such as Anacin and Excedrin, may contain caffeine.

• *Sugar* is bad news for people with anxiety. It's well-known that simple sugars, found in candy, cakes, cookies and ice cream, cause your body to release too much of the blood sugar–reducing hormone insulin. This imbalance leads to a severe drop in blood sugar that causes many people to feel light-headed and anxious. But *all* simple sugars—including corn syrup, fructose and honey—may have this effect.

What your body really needs is complex carbohydrates to burn as energy-producing fuel. Good sources include unrefined grains, found in cereal...vegetables, such as asparagus and avocados (both are rich sources of stress-reducing vitamin B)...and fresh fruit.

• *Salt* does more than raise blood pressure in some people. It causes the body to excrete potassium, which helps keep your nervous system healthy.

Read food labels to minimize your sodium intake, and avoid salting your food. Instead, use a natural salt substitute, such as tamari (available at specialty-food stores), or lemon or herbs, especially basil and oregano, for seasoning.

GET THE RIGHT MINERALS...

• *Calcium* acts as a natural tranquilizer. People who are calcium deficient often suffer from heart palpitations, insomnia and nervousness. To increase your dietary intake of calcium, eat more sardines, tofu, broccoli, kale, Chinese cabbage, etc.

• *Magnesium* works with calcium to relieve anxiety. People who are magnesium deficient often experience nervousness, irritability and weakness. Magnesium-rich foods include halibut, avocados and almonds.

Eating a diet rich in the minerals potassium (salmon, cod and apricots)...zinc (whole grains, kidney beans and chickpeas)... and phosphorus (oat bran, chicken and sunflower seeds) is also important for alleviating anxiety. To ensure adequate mineral intake, take a multimineral supplement.

USE GENTLE HERBS...

Because herbs can be as powerful as drugs and sometimes interact with prescription medication, I recommend those with the best safety records. Tell your health-care practitioner which herbs you are taking.

• *Chamomile* is a mild relaxant. Drink a cup of chamomile tea before bed or during a "coffee break." Start with one to two cups daily. Do *not* use this herb if you're allergic to plants of the daisy family.

• *Peppermint leaf* calms the nerves. Drink one cup of peppermint leaf tea after meals to help with digestion and promote relaxation.

• *Nutmeg* promotes sleep, which often is disrupted in people with anxiety. For best results, grind one whole nutmeg in a coffee grinder and place the powdered herb in empty capsules, which you can buy at health-food stores. Keep the capsules in the refrigerator and use within one week. As a sleep aid, take one nutmeg capsule four to five hours before bedtime. For daytime anxiety, take one capsule in the morning.

EXERCISE EVERY DAY...

Exercise provides an ideal outlet for your body when you're exposed to excessive adrenaline due to stress. By triggering the release of "feel-good" chemicals known as endorphins, physical activity acts as a natural tranquilizer.

Everyone knows the benefits of exercise—but few people do it daily. Thirty minutes a day is ideal. If you have difficulty scheduling this, break your activity into three 10-minute sessions or two 15-minute workouts. You don't have to go to a gym—climb up and down some nearby stairs, garden or take a brisk walk at lunchtime.

To successfully integrate physical activity into your daily life, don't do the same thing all the time—instead, mix it up. For example, try activities like swimming...yoga...weight-lifting...

team sports...and dancing. The more variety, the more likely you are to stick to an exercise program.

CREATE NEW HABITS...

Anxiety can encourage people to adopt bad habits, such as drinking too much alcohol and/or smoking. Do whatever you must to stop these behaviors—go to Alcoholics Anonymous, use a smoking-cessation program, etc. Subtle habits—ones that you might not realize are harmful—also contribute to anxiety.

• *Living with negative "self-talk."* Indoctrination from as far back as childhood can make for an anxious adult.

THINK BACK: Were you taught unhealthy beliefs, such as "Life is dangerous" or "I must be perfect?" Do your best to change these beliefs and replace them with affirmations.

EXAMPLES: "I am becoming more relaxed"..."I believe in myself"..."I can relax and breathe calmly." By replacing negative thoughts that cause tension with more positive ones that calm you, anxiety is reduced.

• *Not being assertive enough.* If you tend to do too much for family members and/or friends, learn to say "no." This may be easier said than done. That's why I often recommend taking a course in assertiveness training. Call your community college or look in your local newspaper to find a course near you.

Lack of assertiveness causes people to hold in feelings, which allows anxiety to mount. Assertiveness allows you to say what is on your mind in a constructive and respectful way, which reduces the tension associated with anxiety.

• *Accepting bad relationships.* Many times, family members and/or friends mean well but replicate old patterns that create anxiety. Speak to them about your anxiety. If they don't make changes that help relieve your discomfort, avoid these people whenever you can.

If they are binding relationships, it is important to seek out therapy or learn self-help skills, such as total body relaxation or imagery, to learn how to cope.

Diet and lifestyle changes should relieve some anxiety within a few days. Assertiveness skills may take longer. If you don't get adequate relief, seek counseling with a mental health professional or a counselor skilled in behavioral change.

■

REPORT #54

HELP FOR HEADACHES

Source: **Robert B. Daroff, MD,** professor of neurology and associate dean at Case Western Reserve University School of Medicine, Cleveland. He also is chief of staff and senior vice president for academic affairs at University Hospitals of Cleveland and president of the American Headache Society.

When a patient complains of headache, most doctors simply pull out their prescription pads.

Fortunately, researchers have recently discovered new approaches to preventing and treating this all-too-common condition.

Headache specialist Robert B. Daroff, MD, helped organize a gathering of hundreds of prominent headache researchers who discussed new scientific findings during the American Headache Society's annual meeting in Chicago. **LATEST DEVELOPMENTS...**

BETTER MIGRAINE DETECTION...

Fewer than half of the estimated 30 million Americans who suffer from migraine receive an accurate diagnosis. Patients—and their doctors—often mistake it for a tension or sinus headache. Because treatments that may be effective for these conditions aren't effective for migraine, a missed diagnosis often leads to unnecessary discomfort and frustration.

Headache experts have no trouble recognizing migraines. That's primarily because they typically take an hour to evaluate each new patient. Primary-care physicians don't have the time—or, in some cases, the expertise—to properly identify migraine symptoms.

NEW STUDY: Researchers at the Albert Einstein College of Medicine in New York City gave a simple survey to 443 patients with a history of headache. **MORE THAN 90% OF THOSE WHO ANSWERED "YES" TO TWO OF THREE KEY QUESTIONS WERE FOUND TO HAVE MIGRAINES...**

• *Has a headache limited your activities* for one or more days in the last three months?

• *Are you nauseated* when you have a headache?

• *Does light bother you* when you have a headache?

IMPLICATION: The three-question test provides a quick, accurate guideline that can help primary-care physicians make a proper diagnosis.

The test isn't a perfect diagnostic tool. For example, some people who answer "yes" to two of the questions may turn out to have an underlying disease, such as cancer.

CAUTION: Patients as well as doctors frequently confuse migraine with chronic sinusitis. But migraine symptoms—intense pain along with nausea and/or visual disturbances, such as auras, in the absence of fever—are almost never caused by sinus infection.

HERBS AND HEADACHE...

Nearly half of all Americans use herbal remedies on occasion. This includes ginkgo biloba for circulation...ginseng for energy...echinacea for colds...St. John's wort for depression... garlic supplements for heart health, etc. What most people don't realize is that some of these common herbs can actually trigger headache or interact with conventional headache treatments.

NEW STUDY: University of Utah researchers identified the herbal products that are most commonly used in the US. The researchers then scoured the scientific literature and identified possible side effects and/or potential drug interactions.

THEIR FINDINGS...

Ginkgo biloba, ginseng, echinacea, St. John's wort and garlic supplements interfere with liver enzymes that break down the migraine drug *sumatriptan* (Imitrex) and the tricyclic antidepressants *amitriptyline* (Elavil) and *nortriptyline* (Aventyl), which are also commonly used for migraine prevention and treatment.

POSSIBLE RESULT: Dangerous drug levels can accumulate in the bloodstream.

Combining herbs with drugs may also make treatments less effective, causing your doctor to prescribe unnecessarily high doses.

Ginkgo biloba may even cause headache in some people.

IMPLICATION: Patients undergoing treatment for migraine or cluster headache should *not* take ginkgo biloba, ginseng, echinacea, St. John's wort or garlic supplements without the supervision of their physician.

Because over-the-counter (OTC) analgesics taken at the onset of a headache do not always relieve symptoms, some patients take these drugs daily. But the long-term daily use of such medication increases the risk for side effects, such as gastric irritation or bleeding.

In addition, daily use of OTC or prescription drugs can cause severe *rebound* headaches—chronic daily headaches that occur when medication wears off.

BOTOX AND HEADACHE...

NEW STUDY: Researchers at Kaiser Permanente in San Diego gave injections of *botulinum toxin* (Botox), the popular antiwrinkle treatment, to 271 headache patients who failed to get relief from standard treatments. Patients in the study were given injections every three months, for a period of six to 15 months.

At the conclusion of the study, 80% of participants said their headaches were less frequent, less intense or both. About 95% reported no side effects. This study, the largest to date on Botox and headaches, confirms the results of previous studies.

Most patients get 30 small injections per treatment, usually in areas of the scalp where pain is present.

IMPLICATION: Botox reduces the frequency of headaches and is a good choice for sufferers who don't get relief from other methods. The use of Botox for headaches is still experimental, so insurance will not pay for it.

BENEFITS OF COUNSELING...

The debilitating pain of migraine affects emotional as well as physical health. It's common for people who get frequent migraines to feel frustrated or be misunderstood by friends and colleagues who fail to appreciate the degree of their discomfort. Although doctors routinely treat physical symptoms, they often don't give sufficient attention to the emotional components of chronic headache pain.

NEW STUDY: Ohio University researchers gave more than 100 migraine patients a battery of psychological and neurological tests. Nearly one-third of them were found to have mood or anxiety disorders. Depression was the most common diagnosis, followed by generalized anxiety disorder.

People who suffer frequent migraines understandably get depressed and anxious, but migraines are *not* the cause. It's possible that there's a third, underlying factor—possibly an imbalance in serotonin or other neurotransmitters—that triggers migraine as well as mood disorders.

IMPLICATION: Migraines and other kinds of chronic pain are frequently accompanied by depression and/or anxiety. Patients who are depressed tend to experience even more pain. They're also less likely to pursue positive coping strategies, such as exercise or healthful dietary changes.

All migraine patients should consider seeing a therapist for psychotherapy and/or medication to help them cope with the psychological stress associated with migraine headaches.

REPORT #55

WHICH FOODS HELP EASE CHRONIC FATIGUE SYMPTOMS?

Source: **Basant K. Puri, MD, PhD,** consultant and senior lecturer, Imperial College, University of London. His study was published in *Acta Psychiatrica Scandinavica*, Skovagervej 2, DK-8240 Risskov, Denmark.

Chronic fatigue syndrome, a condition characterized by fatigue and musculoskeletal pain, is linked to an imbalance of *phospholipids*, a type of fat, in the brain. *Eicosapentaenoic acid* (EPA), a fat found in fish, restores that balance by inhibiting the breakdown of phospholipids and helping form new ones. Eating more salmon, white albacore tuna and other fatty fish rich in EPA may ease the fatigue and depression often associated with this condition. Consult your doctor about the best way to incorporate this dietary strategy into your treatment plan.

REPORT #56

VITAMIN C CAN HELP YOU PERK UP

Source: **Carol Johnston, PhD,** professor of nutrition, Arizona State University, Tempe. Her study of 494 people was published in the *Journal of the American College of Nutrition,* Wayne State University, 5057 Woodward, Detroit 48202.

Feelings of general fatigue may be caused by a lack of vitamin C. A study of fatigued but otherwise healthy adults found that 30% were depleted of this antioxidant vitamin. Six percent had levels of vitamin C so low that they were at risk of developing scurvy. In addition to fatigue, vitamin C deficiency can cause joint pain, bleeding gums and/or a rash on the lower legs. Foods high in vitamin C include oranges, broccoli and cantaloupe.

REPORT #57

THE HEARTBURN CURE THAT WON'T HOLLOW YOUR BONES

Source: **Mark A. Stengler, ND,** naturopathic physician in private practice, La Jolla, CA...associate clinical professor at the National College of Naturopathic Medicine, Portland, OR...author of numerous books, including *The Natural Physician's Healing Therapies* and coauthor of *Prescription for Natural Cures* (both from Bottom Line Books)...and author of the *Bottom Line/Natural Healing* newsletter.

Up to 18% of Americans experience heartburn at least once weekly. Heartburn that occurs more than twice a week may be gastroesophageal reflux disease (GERD), a condition in which stomach contents back up into the esophagus. The most commonly prescribed drugs for heartburn and GERD are *esomeprazole* (Nexium), *lansoprazole* (Prevacid), *rabeprazole* (Aciphex), *omeprazole* (Prilosec) and *pantoprazole* (Protonix).

Known as proton pump inhibitors (PPIs), these drugs block the production of stomach acid. And they carry a hefty price tag—about $4 per dose. Potential side effects include diarrhea, vomiting, headache, rash, dizziness, abnormal heartbeat, muscle pain, leg cramps and water retention. In one study, subjects taking a heartburn drug experienced a 41% to 61% drop in calcium absorption.

NATURAL ALTERNATIVES...

Try them in this order—each one alone—for two weeks at a time until you find what works effectively for you. You can take more than one at a time.

CAUTION: Do *not* stop taking a prescription drug or begin using a supplement unless you are being monitored by a health professional.

Natural alternatives work best when combined with diet and lifestyle improvements, particularly regular exercise, stress-reduction techniques and adequate sleep.

• *Licorice root* (in chewable wafers or powder form) reduces heartburn and irritation of the digestive tract lining. Take 500 milligrams (mg) to 1,000 mg three times daily 30 minutes before meals.

A special type of licorice root, known as deglycyrrhizinated licorice (DGL), does not elevate blood pressure, as do some varieties of the herb. DGL is widely available at health-food stores and pharmacies. It should relieve your symptoms within two weeks. Take as needed if symptoms recur.

• *Nux vomica,* a homeopathic remedy derived from the seeds of the poison nut tree, has helped many of my patients reduce or eliminate heartburn. It soothes irritation of the digestive lining and is believed to help the upper esophageal valve close more efficiently, thereby preventing reflux. Take two 30C potency pellets three times daily until your symptoms are eliminated. Improvement should occur within two weeks. Resume treatment if symptoms return.

Because nux vomica is also used to treat asthma, it is good for asthmatics who suffer from heartburn.

• *Aloe vera,* a cactus-like member of the lily family, soothes and promotes healing of the lining of the digestive tract. Some people who don't respond to DGL get relief from aloe vera. Drink one-quarter cup of aloe vera juice or take a 500-mg capsule three times daily.

REPORT #58

THE HEALING POWER OF WATER

Source: **Dian Dincin Buchman, PhD,** a New York City–based lecturer on water therapy and other alternative therapies. She is author of several books, including *The Complete Book of Water Healing.* McGraw-Hill.

Ice packs, hot and cold compresses, medicated baths and other forms of water therapy were mainstays of folk medicine for centuries.

Today, high-tech medicine has eclipsed water-based treatments. Yet these treatments—safe, inexpensive and easy to use—remain valuable tools for easing discomfort caused by common ailments.

MEDICATED BATHS...

We all know how relaxing a warm bath can be. But not everyone realizes that even *greater* benefits can be reaped by adding natural ingredients to the water.

• *Apple cider vinegar.* Add a cup to bathwater, and splash a handful over your shoulders, back and chest. That will invigorate you when you're fatigued.

This technique also helps restore the skin's germ-killing natural acidity, which is continually washed away by bathing.

To soothe poison ivy or sunburn, add *two* cups of vinegar.

• *Bran.* A bran bath eases itching, soothes dermatitis or other skin irritations and eliminates scaly patches.

Sew several handfuls of wheat or oat bran into a cheesecloth pouch. Soak the pouch in hot water for several minutes, then place in a tub filled with tepid water. Squeeze the pouch until the water turns milky.

• *Pine extract.* One capful in a warm bath helps open clogged pores, speeds healing of rashes and relieves muscle fatigue.

Pine extract is available at many drugstores and health-food stores. Do not confuse it with pine *cleanser*, which will irritate the skin.

SALT MASSAGE...

This energizing technique tones tissues, relieves stress and fatigue...and can help you ward off a cold.

Sit on the edge of a tub filled with warm water. Pour salt into a cupped hand. Slowly add water to the salt until you make a thick paste.

Using firm, circular motions, rub the paste over your body. Then rinse off the paste with a soak in the tub...or sponge it off with cold water. Be careful not to rub salt onto sores, cuts, etc.

HAND BATH...

To ease writer's cramp, soak hands in hot water. To warm cold hands, soak them alternately in hot water (three minutes) and cold water (30 seconds). Repeat several times, ending with cold water.

CAUTION: Don't leave hands in cold water for more than a few minutes at a time.

COLD-WATER TREADING...

Fill the tub ankle-deep with cold water. Holding on to a firmly anchored rail, march in place for a few seconds or minutes (as long as you can comfortably tolerate). Then rub your feet briskly with a towel.

Done twice daily, this technique creates a remarkable sense of well-being...and is great for relieving exercise-related leg cramps. Some believe that it builds resistance to disease.

Done at night, cold-water treading promotes sound sleep— yet it has an eye-opening effect when done in the morning.

COMPRESSES...

To prevent or relieve headache pain, fold a washcloth in half, dip it in ice water and wring it out. Place it on your head or neck. Rewet it every few minutes to keep it cold.

To relieve a sore throat or laryngitis, fold a cotton cloth in thirds, wet it with cold water and wring it out. Wind it once around the neck and fasten with a safety pin. Over the cloth, wrap a wool scarf.

Leave this wrap in place as long as you like. With the cold trapped against the skin by the wool, the body continues to divert more warming blood to the area—helping break up congestion.

REPORT #59

USE COLD-WATER THERAPY
FOR RELIEF

Source: **Alexa Fleckenstein, MD,** board-certified internist who practices traditional and complementary medicine. Dr. Fleckenstein holds a German subspecialty degree in natural medicine.

For most Americans, a steaming-hot bath or shower is a daily routine. But for more than 150 years, numerous Europeans have used invigorating *cold* showers and swims to promote good health.

Scientific evidence and numerous case histories support the use of "cold-water therapy" as an adjunct to standard treatments for frequent colds, insomnia, high blood pressure—even cancer and other serious disorders.

HOW IT BEGAN...

Cold-water therapy was first popularized in Germany by the priest Sebastian Kneipp (1821–1897). In the winter of 1849, Kneipp successfully battled then-incurable tuberculosis by plunging several times weekly into the frigid Danube River. His 1886 book, *My Water Cure*, became an international best-seller.

THE MECHANISM...

When practiced for at least four weeks, cold-water therapy...

• *Stabilizes blood pressure.* Cold water triggers the autonomic nervous system—which controls involuntary functions, such as heartbeat and breathing—to raise blood pressure, increase heart rate and constrict blood vessels.

The autonomic responses strengthen with each exposure. This stabilizes blood pressure, improves circulation and balances other bodily functions, such as the sleep/wake cycle.

• *Enhances immunity.* Cold water triggers the release of cytokines and other hormone-like substances that are key to improving immune function.

RECENT FINDING: Breast cancer patients who underwent cold-water therapy for four weeks experienced significant gains in their levels of disease-fighting white blood cells, according to a German study.

• *Reduces pain.* Cold causes the body to release *endorphins*, hormones with proven pain-fighting properties.

• *Improves moods.* Cold water activates sensory nerves that lead to the brain. A cold, exhilarating shower can be emotionally uplifting and prime a person for new experiences.

THE REGIMEN...

To gain the benefits of cold-water therapy at home, begin with your usual warm shower. When you're finished, step out of the water stream and turn off the hot water. Leave the cold water running.*

Start by wetting your feet first. Next, expose the hands and face to the cold water.

IMPORTANT: Jumping in all at once may hinder circulation.

Finally, step under the shower. Let the cold water run over your scalp, face, the front of your body and then down your back. You can begin by taking a cold shower that lasts only a couple of seconds.

After one month, the entire process should last no more than 40 seconds. Work up to whatever is comfortable for you.

IF YOU CAN'T TOLERATE THE COLD: Keep the water cold but expose only your feet, hands and face. Gradually increase the duration and area of exposure.

CAUTION: People who are very thin or frail may be unable to tolerate cold showers in the beginning. If you do not feel warm and invigorated after the shower, decrease the length of your next cold shower.

If you still don't feel warm within minutes, forgo cold showers. Instead, condition your body with cold sponge baths of the feet, hands, face—and then the rest of your body—after your warm shower.

Do not try cold-water therapy if you suffer from an acute illness, such as severe back pain...have hardening of the arteries (*atherosclerosis*)...Raynaud's disease...or have high blood pressure not controlled by medication.

Cold water causes a spike in blood pressure, which can be dangerous for those with conditions such as unmanaged hypertension.

*Water temperature should be about 60°F. In all but the hottest areas, water straight from the cold faucet will do. If your water is not cold enough to give you a good jolt, enhance the effect by air-drying—rather than towel-drying—your body.

The therapy can be safely used to reduce mildly elevated blood pressure (150/100 and below) or to raise low blood pressure.

IF YOU HAVE QUESTIONS ABOUT YOUR BLOOD PRESSURE: See your doctor for a blood pressure test before starting a cold-water regimen.

■

REPORT #60

THE 3-MINUTE PAIN-ERASING MIRACLE

Source: **Joseph Weisberg, PhD,** a physical therapist and dean of Touro College School of Health Sciences in New York City and Bay Shore, and founder and owner of North Shore Rehabilitation in Great Neck, all in NY. He is coauthor of *3 Minutes to a Pain-Free Life*. Atria.

Conventional treatments for chronic pain, such as medication and surgery, mainly aim to relieve pain symptoms, including spasm and inflammation—but often do not address the *cause* of the pain. That's like applying grease to squeaky shock absorbers on a car. The noise may disappear temporarily, but the underlying problem is still there—and the squeaks return.

GOOD NEWS: Most chronic pain can be prevented—or relieved—with a movement therapy program. Unlike drugs, surgery or other conventional treatments, this approach corrects the causes of pain by lengthening muscles and allowing joints to move through their full range of motion.

UNDERLYING CAUSES OF PAIN...

Few cases of chronic musculoskeletal pain are due to serious injuries.

MAIN CAUSE: A sedentary lifestyle. The body's muscles and joints must be moved through their full range to remain stretched and lubricated.

However, most Americans remain inactive for long periods of time while at work, watching television, etc. As a result, muscle fibers shorten and joint movement becomes limited. Common, unavoidable positions and movements, such as sitting, reaching, gripping and bending over, cause *microtraumas* to muscles— minute tears that are so subtle that they cause no pain initially and fail to trigger the body's healing mechanisms.

After years or decades, these microtraumas accumulate and cause pain. Patients begin to curtail their normal range of motion—taking shorter steps, getting up slowly from chairs, not bending down, etc.—to minimize discomfort.

THERAPEUTIC MOVEMENTS...

Most people can reverse this cycle with a program of six 30-second exercises that target the musculoskeletal system.* Performed daily for a total of only three minutes, these movements increase joint lubrication and lengthen and strengthen muscle fibers. This reduces your likelihood of developing microtraumas, thus eliminating the underlying causes of most chronic pain.

BOW...

PRIMARY AREAS WORKED: Spine, shoulders, hips, knees and ankles.

HOW IT HELPS: The spine is essential to most common movements, including standing, sitting, bending and raising and lowering the head. However, the spine is rarely taken through its full range of motion. The Bow mobilizes all of the spinal joints and stretches the paraspinal muscles—layers of muscles that run along the spine and are involved in most cases of back pain.

WHAT TO DO: Kneel on the floor, and sit back on your heels. Bend over and reach your arms as far forward as you can. Place your palms flat on the floor, arms shoulder-width apart and fingers spread out. Hold for 30 seconds.

ARCH...

PRIMARY AREAS WORKED: Spine, neck, wrists, hands, fingers and abdomen.

HOW IT HELPS: This movement also targets the spine and takes the neck through its full range of motion. The movement

*Check with your doctor before beginning this—or any—exercise program.

of arching both upward and downward causes the abdominal muscles to contract and then relax, strengthening these muscles to better stabilize and support the lower back.

WHAT TO DO: Begin in a kneeling position, with your palms flat on the floor under your shoulders. Spread 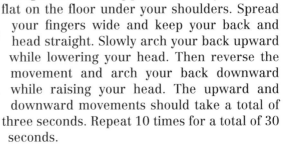 your fingers wide and keep your back and head straight. Slowly arch your back upward while lowering your head. Then reverse the movement and arch your back downward while raising your head. The upward and downward movements should take a total of three seconds. Repeat 10 times for a total of 30 seconds.

LIZARD...

PRIMARY AREAS WORKED: Spine (especially spinal discs) and lower back.

HOW IT HELPS: Disc problems are among the main causes of chronic pain. Prolonged sitting and frequent bending can cause discs in the lower back to bulge or rupture (herniate). The Lizard extends the spine and can push discs back into their normal positions.

WHAT TO DO: Lie on your stomach. Place your palms flat on the floor, slightly more than shoulder-width apart. Flex your 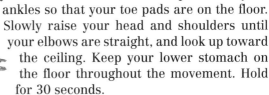 ankles so that your toe pads are on the floor. Slowly raise your head and shoulders until your elbows are straight, and look up toward the ceiling. Keep your lower stomach on the floor throughout the movement. Hold for 30 seconds.

IMPORTANT: If the movement causes pain, modify it by not quite straightening your elbows, which will reduce the stretch.

NATURAL SQUAT...

PRIMARY AREAS WORKED: Lower back and pelvis.

HOW IT HELPS: Sitting is among the main causes of back, leg and hip pain. The Natural Squat stretches the entire lower back...reduces pressure on the spinal discs...and stretches the pelvis, hips, knees and ankles.

WHAT TO DO: With your feet shoulder-width apart, squat down, keeping your heels flat on the floor. You can wrap your arms around your knees or hold them straight in front of you. Hold for 30 seconds.

SPLIT...

PRIMARY AREAS WORKED: Hips, inner thighs, groin and knees.

HOW IT HELPS: The hips are designed to abduct (move the legs away from the body), but this movement is rarely performed in daily life. The inner thigh muscles are also underutilized. The Split works the inner thigh and groin muscles and stretches the hamstring (back of thigh) muscles. Strengthening and stretching these muscles reduces knee and hip strain and injury.

WHAT TO DO: While standing, spread your legs as far as you comfortably can while keeping the feet parallel and knees straight. Hold this position for 15 seconds. Then, bending at the waist, lean forward as far as you can, keeping your knees straight. Your hands may touch the floor, but they don't have to. Hold for 15 seconds.

SKY REACH...

PRIMARY AREAS WORKED: Spine, shoulders, forearms, elbows, wrists, hands and fingers.

HOW IT HELPS: The Sky Reach improves posture. It also works muscles in the upper extremities, including the rotator cuffs in the shoulders. These are among the most-used muscles in the body—and most prone to injury. The forearm muscles, which support the elbows, hands and fingers, are also stretched. And the wrists are exercised in their full range of motion.

WHAT TO DO: Sit on the floor with your legs comfortably crossed. Interlace the fingers of your hands. Keeping your back straight, lift your arms up and over your head. With palms facing upward, reach as high as you can. Hold for 30 seconds.

Illustrations by Shawn Banner.

REPORT #61

THE "MINERAL CURE" FOR CANCER

Source: **Mark A. Stengler, ND,** naturopathic physician in private practice, La Jolla, CA…associate clinical professor at the National College of Naturopathic Medicine, Portland, OR…author of numerous books, including *The Natural Physician's
Healing Therapies* and coauthor of *Prescription for Natural Cures* (both from Bottom
Line Books)…and author of the *Bottom Line/Natural Healing* newsletter.

Selenium is a trace mineral that plays an important role in many functions of the body. Brazil nuts are one of the best sources of selenium. It is also found in Brewer's yeast, wheat germ, whole grains, broccoli, red grapes, onions, garlic, egg yolks, red meat, chicken and seafood. The amount of selenium in plant foods vary depending on the area of the country (or world) in which they're grown. Since a selenium deficiency can compromise one's health, the use of supplementation makes good preventive sense—but don't take more than 600 micrograms a day.

Selenium is a necessary nutrient that helps your immune system function more efficiently. It has been shown to stimulate the activity of white blood cells, the key players involved in fighting infections and cancer. It is also a critical component of your body's antioxidant system, which defends against harmful molecules known as free radicals.

Selenium supplements are used therapeutically for conditions such as AIDS, arthritis (rheumatoid and osteoarthritis), cataracts, depression, cancer prevention, heart attack prevention, hepatitis C and hypothyroidism; it also improves sperm motility.

Preliminary studies have shown that selenium helps reduce the risk of certain types of cancer, including prostate cancer. In one study, it was discovered that men who consumed the most selenium in their diet developed 65% fewer cases of advanced prostate cancer than did men with the lowest levels of selenium intake. Another eye-opening study conducted at the University of Arizona in Tucson looked at the effect of selenium supplementation on patients with a history of basal or squamous cell skin cancer. The study involved a total of 1,312 patients, with an average age of 63 years. For almost three years, patients were given either 200 micrograms of selenium supplements or a placebo. Researchers found significant reductions in total cancer mortality (29 deaths in the selenium treatment group and 57 deaths in the control group), as well as total cancer incidence (77 cancers in the selenium group and 119 in the control group). Selenium supplementation provided a significant reduction in the incidence of lung, colorectal and prostate cancers.

To help prevent cancer, the best source of selenium is from Brewer's yeast.

REPORT #62

NATURAL DECONGESTANT

> *Source:* **Sanford M. Archer, MD,** associate professor of otolaryngology, University of Kentucky Chandler Medical Center, Lexington.

To quickly unstuff your nose, sniff horseradish. It contains *allyl isothiocyanate*, a compound similar to the active ingredient in decongestants. Take a sniff two or three times daily. Keep your nose six inches from the jar, and don't spread your germs by breathing directly onto it. Better yet, keep a separate jar for decongestant purposes.

CAUTION: If sinus congestion lasts for more than a week, or is accompanied by green mucus, postnasal drip, pain or toothache, be sure to see your doctor.

REPORT #63

"PAT'S CURE" FOR CHRONIC SINUS TROUBLE

> *Source:* **Mark A. Stengler, ND,** naturopathic physician in private practice, La Jolla, CA...associate clinical professor at the National College of Naturopathic Medicine, Portland, OR...author of numerous books, including *The Natural Physician's Healing Therapies* and coauthor of *Prescription for Natural Cures* (both from Bottom Line Books)...and author of the *Bottom Line/Natural Healing* newsletter.

An estimated 37 million Americans suffer from sinusitis each year, and nearly 32 million cases of chronic sinusitis are reported annually. If you're one of these people, you know what it feels like to have repeated bouts of sinus swelling and infections, tenderness in the face, aching behind the eyes and difficulty breathing through the nose. Most sinus sufferers I see have taken antibiotics and a host of allergy medications for years, and they finally have grown tired of these temporary fixes. I help these people by treating the underlying causes of chronic sinusitis with natural, nontoxic therapies.

A MISSING LINK...

One important root cause of sinusitis that is rarely addressed by conventional physicians is fungus. The dark, moist sinus cavities are a great environment for fungus growth. An overgrowth or infection of fungal microbes is most likely to occur after repeated use of antibiotics and steroidal nasal sprays, which suppress the localized immune response.

In 1999, researchers at the Mayo Clinic announced to the medical community that fungus was a primary cause of sinusitis. Their first study involved 210 patients with chronic sinusitis. Using new, more accurate methods of testing, which included evaluating immune and allergy reactions to fungus with a special type of nasal swab, the researchers discovered fungus in the nasal mucus of 96% of the patients.

They also identified 40 different kinds of fungus in these people, with an average of 2.7 kinds per person. According to David Sherris, MD, one of the primary researchers, "Our studies indicate that, in fact, fungus is likely the cause of nearly all of these problems. And it is not an allergic reaction, but an immune reaction." In another Mayo Clinic study, all 54 participants who had a history of chronic sinusitis tested positive for fungus.

When the sinus cavities are overrun with fungi, the body responds by marshaling immune cells, such as *T-lymphocytes* and *eosinophils*, for an attack. This results in irritation and inflammation of the sinus membranes.

HOW TREATMENT GOES AWRY...

Despite all the information from the prestigious Mayo Clinic (which also was given a $2.5 million National Institutes of Health grant to further investigate the mechanisms behind this immunologic response to the fungi), many doctors—including ear, nose and throat (ENT) specialists—still don't address fungal overgrowth and fungal sensitivity in patients suffering from chronic sinusitis. In fact, many doctors continue to prescribe therapies, such as steroidal nasal sprays, that actually *promote* fungal overgrowth.

Almost every patient with chronic sinusitis who has come to my office had been prescribed a steroidal nasal spray. One of the most widely used is *fluticasone* (Flonase), which contains a synthetic corticosteroid that reduces inflammation in the nasal passageways and sinuses. Similar steroidal sprays include *triamcinolone* (Nasacort) and *mometasone* (Nasonex). Ironically, the package insert for Flonase lists one of its potential side effects as an overgrowth of the fungus *Candida albicans* in the sinus and throat!

Here's an interesting case from my practice. Pat, a 49-year-old woman with a chronic sinus problem, had been given more than 25 courses of antibiotics over the past 10 years. She also had used various allergy and sinus medications, including Flonase and the steroid *prednisone*, which also is known to set the stage for fungal overgrowth.

When Pat came to my office, I recommended an antifungal treatment program consisting of a grapefruit seed extract nasal spray, an herbal product containing a strong dose of oregano oil and a probiotic containing *acidophilus* and *bifidobacterium*.

I also suggested natural anti-inflammatories for her sinuses, including the flavonoid *quercetin* and a protease enzyme. (I'll describe the mechanism for each therapy below.) Within four weeks, Pat's symptoms dramatically improved, and she has been antibiotic-free ever since.

OTHER CULPRITS...

If you suffer from sinusitis, it's important to make sure that there's no structural defect in the nasal passageways or sinuses that hinders drainage. An ENT doctor can order a computed tomography (CT) scan of the sinus and perhaps an X-ray or magnetic resonance imaging (MRI) of the sinus cavity. A structural defect that prevents drainage may require surgery—although I suggest that the patient see more than one ENT specialist to confirm that there is a structural blockage.

Undetected dental infections, including low-grade infections in root canals, can also cause chronic sinusitis. Antibiotics don't always kill such infections, since root canals have poor blood supply and bacteria can become trapped there.

I strongly urge my patients to avoid the long-term use (two weeks or longer) of steroidal nasal sprays. Instead, focus on cleansing the sinus cavities with the following natural antifungal, antiallergy and anti-inflammatory therapies.

NATURAL TREATMENT REGIMEN...

• *Diet.* Consume a diet that is bountiful in vegetables, fruits, nuts, seeds, fresh fish and lean poultry. If you can tolerate them, I also highly recommend adding onions, oregano and garlic liberally to your meals. They all have potent antifungal effects. Flaxseed also has antifungal properties. Mix one to two tablespoons of freshly ground flaxseed daily into your cereal, salad or yogurt. It adds a delicious nutty flavor. Just be sure to drink 10 ounces of water within 30 minutes of eating flaxseed. Otherwise, you can get a blockage in your intestine.

Avoid simple sugar products, such as alcohol, soda, white bread and refined pasta, and have no more than eight ounces a day of any unsweetened fruit juice—they suppress immunity, worsen inflammation and promote the growth of fungus. Finally, be wary of cow's milk and wheat, which often exacerbate sinusitis.

Most people who have chronic sinusitis need to use a combination of natural remedies. For mild cases, try oregano and quercetin. For severe chronic cases or for cases in which oregano and quercetin don't work sufficiently, try all the treatments recommended. Children can follow the dietary suggestions made here, but supplement use should be supervised by a doctor.

• *Oregano oil.* This herbal remedy has been shown to be the most potent available for fungal infections. It should be consumed orally, not put into the nose. I recommend taking it by itself in liquid or capsule form or in a combination herbal formula. North American Herb & Spice (800-444-4584, *www. oregano-oil.net*) has an excellent oregano extract that has been studied by Georgetown University and found to have potent antifungal effects. The liquid version of this combination extract is so potent that you should start by placing two drops under the tongue twice daily and build up to four drops daily over the course of a week. If the taste is too strong, dilute in two to four ounces of water. The recommended dose for the oregano capsule is two to four 250-milligram (mg) capsules daily. If you are prone to heartburn or ulcers, use oregano with caution—the essential oils can irritate some people's digestive tracts.

• *Quercetin.* This nutrient, which has a natural anti-inflammatory and antihistamine effect, belongs to a family of plant chemicals called flavonoids. It is in onions, apples, green and black tea, vegetables and beans. Because allergies are so common with sinusitis, I recommend that my patients take 500 mg of quercetin (in capsule form) twice daily for its anti-inflammatory effects and to reduce allergy symptoms. Quercetin supplements are available at health-food stores and pharmacies.

• *Grapefruit seed extract.* This antifungal/antimicrobial is available in a nasal spray.

TO USE: Tilt your head back and pump once into each nostril. For chronic bacterial and/or fungal infections, use once daily...for acute infections, four times daily. I often recommend NutriBiotic Nasal Spray (800-225-4345, *www.nutribiotic.com*).

• *Probiotics.* "Good" bacteria is a key component in your immune system's ability to keep fungi and other microbes in check. It's important to replenish these bacteria in your sinuses and digestive tract as well as in the rest of your body—it is especially important if you recently used antibiotics, steroidal nasal sprays or the steroid prednisone. Take one pill daily of a probiotic formula containing 3 billion to 5 billion organisms. Good brands include Jarrow (800-726-0886, *www.jarrow. com*) and Bio-K+ (800-593-2465, *www.biokplus.com*)—both available at health-food stores.

• *N-acetylcysteine.* This amino acid–derived nutrient thins mucus and promotes sinus drainage. I recommend 500 mg twice daily for those with acute or chronic sinusitis.

• *Bromelain.* This enzyme, which has a natural anti-inflammatory effect, has been shown to improve acute sinusitis. Protease (protein-digesting) enzyme products also confer this benefit. When treating sinusitis, the key is to take bromelain or protease enzymes between meals to benefit from their anti-inflammatory effect. If you choose a protease enzyme,

Wobenzyme, available online from iHerb.com (866-328-1171, *www.iherb.com*) is a good formula. The dosage is two tablets twice daily between meals. If you choose bromelain, the less expensive option, take 500 mg two times daily between meals.

IMPORTANT: Even though bromelain is made from pineapples, eating pineapple alone does not provide the same benefit because bromelain is taken from the pineapple stem. Bromelain and protease enzymes are available at health-food stores.

CAUTION: Neither protease enzymes nor bromelain should be used if you take a blood thinner, such as *warfarin* (Coumadin), unless supervised by a doctor.

• *Saline rinses.* Saline rinses relieve sinus irritation caused by pollutants, allergens and infections of the nasal passages. Look for a rinse that contains *xylitol*, a natural substance that prevents bacteria from adhering to the nasal cavity. Squirt it in each nostril once or twice a day. Xlear (pronounced "clear") Nasal Wash (877-599-5327, *www.xlear.com*) is a good brand.

REPORT #64

SPICE IT UP TO REDUCE RISK

Source: **Ann W. Hsing, PhD,** investigator, division of cancer epidemiology and genetics, National Cancer Institute, Bethesda, MD. Her study was published in the *Journal of the National Cancer Institute*, 8120 Woodmont Ave., Suite 500, Bethesda, MD 20814.

Eating garlic and chives reduces prostate cancer risk. Members of the *allium* family, garlic and chives are rich in *flavonols*, plant substances known to have antitumor effects. They have previously been shown to help prevent cancer of the stomach, colon and esophagus.

RECENT FINDING: Men who ate 10 grams (g) of these herbs (approximately three cloves of garlic) a day had half the rate of prostate cancer as did men who ate only 2.2 g a day. Onions, leeks and shallots are also beneficial.

REPORT #65

FOODS THAT FIGHT PROSTATE CANCER

Source: **Duane Baldwin**, **MD,** former chief resident urologist, Loma Linda University School of Medicine, Loma Linda, CA. He spoke about prostate cancer at a meeting of the American Urological Association.

It's now clear that a low-fat diet helps prevent prostate cancer. IN ADDITION, CERTAIN FOODS ARE BENEFICIAL...

• *Allicin.* This garlic compound has potent anticancer properties. Add minced garlic to pasta sauces and stir-frys...or you could even toss a peeled clove into the juicer when making fruit juice.

• *Citrus fruits.* Oranges, lemons, etc., are loaded with *pectin*, a fiber that fights cancer. Since most pectin is found in the peels of citrus fruits, try zesting small slices and drizzle them into salads and stir-frys.

• *Gluten.* In a recent study, men who ate gluten-based meat substitutes were two-thirds less likely to have elevated levels of prostate-specific antigen (PSA), a marker for prostate cancer. Try the meat substitute *seitan*, sold in health-food stores and some supermarkets.

• *Omega-3 fatty acids.* In recent studies, men who ate small amounts of omega-3 acids and lots of saturated fat were three times more likely to develop prostate cancer than other men. Omega-3 fatty acids are found in salmon, mackerel and other cold-water fish.

• *Selenium.* In a recent study, men who took selenium supplements had a lower risk for prostate cancer.

GOOD SOURCE OF SELENIUM: Brazil nuts.

• *Soy.* Tofu, tempeh, miso and other soy foods contain *genistein* and other *isoflavones*, compounds that retard the growth of cancer cells. Eat two to three ounces of soy foods a day.

• *Tomatoes.* They're rich in *lycopene*, a pigment that develops anticancer properties once it's been cooked. Make homemade tomato sauce or grill fresh tomatoes.

REPORT #66

FREE SECRET SLASHES PROSTATE CANCER RISK 70%

Source: **Edward L. Giovannucci, MD, ScD,** professor of nutrition and epidemiology, Harvard School of Public Health, Boston.

In a recent finding, men who engaged in at least three hours weekly of vigorous physical activity, such as jogging, swimming or bicycling, had a nearly 70% lower risk of being diagnosed with advanced prostate cancer.

THEORY: Exercise reduces levels of hormones, such as *insulin* and *leptin*, that may contribute to the development of prostate cancer.

FOR OPTIMAL PROSTATE CANCER PREVENTION: Men should aim for at least three hours of vigorous exercise per week. Walking or other types of milder exercise have cardiovascular and other benefits.

■

REPORT #67

SOY FIGHTS PROSTATE CANCER

Source: **Jin-Rong Zhou, PhD,** assistant professor of surgery, Harvard Medical School, Boston.

Compounds in soy called *isoflavones* inhibit the growth and spread of prostate tumors.

HELPFUL: Prostate cancer patients should consume 150 to 200 milligrams (mg) of isoflavones daily. One cup of soy milk contains 20 to 40 mg isoflavones...one-half cup of tofu contains 35 to 40 mg...and one-half cup of soy nuts contains about 170 mg.

IMPORTANT: Check with your doctor before making any changes to your diet.

■

REPORT #68

EATING FISH HELPS, TOO

Source: **Paul Terry, PhD, MPH,** researcher, department of epidemiology and social medicine, Albert Einstein College of Medicine, Bronx, NY.

In one of the first long-term studies of fish consumption and prostate cancer, men who ate little or no fish had up to a three times greater risk for prostate cancer as did men who ate moderate to high amounts of fish. Essential fatty acids in fish seem to inhibit the growth of prostate cancer cells. To achieve this benefit, eat two to three servings of salmon, mackerel, herring or other fatty fish per week.

REPORT #69

SELENIUM VS. PROSTATE CANCER

Source: **James D. Brooks, MD,** assistant professor of urology, Stanford University School of Medicine, Stanford, CA. His study was published in *The Journal of Urology,* 1000 Corporate Blvd., Linthicum, MD 21090.

Men with the lowest levels of selenium were *four times* more likely to develop prostate cancer than those with normal levels, according to a study. Blood levels of this trace element decline with age.

HELPFUL: Men who are age 60 or older should ask their doctor about taking a 200-microgram (mcg) selenium supplement daily. Eating more selenium-rich foods, such as tuna and Brazil nuts, also boosts levels.

REPORT #70

THE ALL-NATURAL CANCER KILLER

Source: **Peter J. Ferguson, PhD,** research associate, London Regional Cancer Program, London, Ontario, Canada.

In laboratory experiments, disease-fighting flavonoids found in cranberries destroyed human prostate cancer cells.

THEORY: Flavonoids interfere with the signals that tell cancer cells to proliferate. More research is under way to confirm these findings. In the meantime, eat homemade cranberry sauce, snack on whole dried cranberries (sold in supermarkets) and/or drink 100% cranberry juice.

■

REPORT #71

PREVENT PROSTATE CANCER NOW

Source: **Sheldon Marks, MD,** adjunct assistant professor of urology at Tufts University School of Medicine in Boston and associate clinical professor of urology and clinical lecturer in radiation oncology at the University of Arizona College of Medicine in Tucson. He is author of *Prostate and Cancer.* Perseus.

When it comes to prostate cancer, doctors have traditionally focused more on treatment than prevention. Depending on the stage of cancer, treatment options include "watchful waiting," surgery or radiation therapy.

Unfortunately, thousands of new cases of prostate cancer are diagnosed in the United States each year, and more than 29,000 American men die from it.

NOW: Promising preventive strategies are being discovered in exciting new research.

EXAMPLE: Recently, researchers at the National Cancer Institute (NCI) reported that healthy men who took the drug *finasteride* (Proscar), which is used to reverse prostate enlargement and male-pattern baldness, had a 25% lower risk of getting prostate cancer than those taking placebos. The study is the first to show that a drug can prevent prostate cancer in a significant number of men.

If you are at high risk for prostate cancer, have a family history of the disease or have an elevated prostate-specific antigen (PSA) reading (above 2.5), ask your doctor if you should take finasteride to help prevent prostate cancer.

Other preventive strategies...

ANTIOXIDANTS...

Cancer starts with damage to DNA or other cell structures. Much of this damage is believed to be triggered by *oxidants* (also called free radicals). These high-energy, oxygen-based molecules are produced by cells during metabolism.

The body naturally produces *antioxidants*, such as *superoxide dismutase*, but not at levels high enough to offset oxidative damage.

Oxidants can be neutralized by eating a diet rich in plant foods. All fruits, vegetables and whole grains contain antioxidant compounds that reduce cell damage as well as the risk for prostate cancer. In some cases, nutritional supplements may be required to get adequate amounts of certain antioxidants.

Examples...

• *Vitamin E.* This antioxidant, which works mainly in the fatty portions of cell membranes, increases immune response and some evidence suggests it decreases the death rate from prostate cancer. You can get some vitamin E from almonds, egg yolks, green, leafy vegetables and vegetable oils, but not enough to protect against prostate cancer.

HELPFUL: Ask your doctor about taking a daily supplement that provides 400 to 800 international units (IU) of vitamin E.

• *Indoles.* These compounds are a derivative of the essential amino acid tryptophan. According to preliminary research conducted at the University of California at Berkeley, the body converts indoles into a substance that guards against prostate cancer growth.

HELPFUL: Eat one to two daily servings of indole-rich cruciferous vegetables, such as brussels sprouts, broccoli or kale.

• *Lycopene.* This plant pigment gives tomatoes and other vegetables their red color. This antioxidant also appears to slow the growth of cancer cells, especially those found in prostate malignancies.

HELPFUL: Eat one to two servings every day of lycopene-rich tomato sauce, tomato paste or ketchup. Processing concentrates the lycopene content.

In addition to tomatoes, other good sources of lycopene include watermelon, red grapefruit and guava.

Don't bother taking lycopene supplements. There's no proof that they work as well as the lycopene in foods.

• *Selenium.* This trace mineral is a powerful antioxidant that also improves the immune system's ability to recognize and destroy cancer cells. Preliminary studies suggest that selenium supplements can help prevent colon and lung malignancies as well as prostate cancer.

HELPFUL: Ask your doctor about taking a nutritional supplement that provides 200 micrograms (mcg) of selenium daily. Although selenium is typically found in Brazil nuts and grains, modern farming methods have depleted large amounts of selenium from the food supply. Selenium is also found in seafood, such as tuna.

FAT CONSUMPTION...

The saturated fat in animal products, such as meat, milk, cheese and many processed foods, not only increases the risk of getting prostate cancer, but also accelerates cancer growth. This is possibly because excess dietary fat stimulates the production of testosterone and testosterone-like hormones, which have been linked to prostate malignancies.

HELPFUL: Don't worry about fat percentages. Instead, simply cut back on your saturated fat consumption.

EXAMPLES: Limit meat to two weekly servings...drink skim or 1% milk instead of 2% or whole milk...cut back on baked goods...increase your intake of fruits and vegetables to replace fat in the diet...and increase your intake of healthy fat, such as omega-3 fatty acids found in salmon, tuna and other cold-water fatty fish.

SOY...

Soy contains estrogen-like plant compounds called *phytoestrogens* that reduce levels of *dihydrotestosterone* (DHT), a steroid hormone that stimulates the development and growth of prostate cancer. Soy may also block *angiogenesis*, the growth of blood vessels that feed tumors.

HELPFUL: Eat two to three weekly servings of tofu, tempeh or other soy foods. Do *not* take soy supplements. They may not guard against prostate cancer as effectively as soy foods, which also contain beneficial vitamins and minerals.

SUN EXPOSURE...

The fear of getting skin cancer has led many American men to avoid sunshine altogether—but doing so could increase their risk for other types of cancer, including prostate. The incidence of prostate cancer is greater in areas in the northwest US and Canada, where there's little sunshine, probably because the body needs ultraviolet light for vitamin D synthesis. Vitamin D helps block the growth of cancer cells.

HELPFUL: Get about 10 minutes of sun exposure without sunscreen daily. If that isn't possible, eat vitamin D–fortified foods, such as milk and breakfast cereals, or ask your doctor about taking a vitamin D supplement.

■

REPORT #72

THE EASY SECRET OF CANCER-PROOF BURGERS

Source: **J. Scott Smith, PhD,** professor, Animal Sciences & Industry, Food Science Institute, Kansas State University, Manhattan, KS.

Spices fight cancer. Research has found that adding fresh rosemary leaves to ground beef lowered the production of cancer-causing compounds during cooking by up to 60%.

THEORY: Antioxidants in rosemary reduce levels of *heterocyclic amines*, known carcinogens found in protein-rich meat that has been grilled, broiled or fried. Basil, oregano and thyme also are believed to confer this benefit.

■

REPORT #73

CANCER FIGHTER ON A SANDWICH

Source: **Paul Talalay, MD,** professor of pharmacology and molecular sciences, Johns Hopkins University School of Medicine, Baltimore.

Broccoli sprouts are rich in a compound that provides significant protection against breast and colon cancers. Sprouts grown from certain broccoli seeds contain up to 50 times more of this compound—*sulforaphane glucosinolate* (SGS)—than mature broccoli. But be aware that the amount of SGS in broccoli sprouts varies widely.

REPORT #74

RAISINS SHRINK COLON CANCER RISK

Source: **Gene Spiller, PhD,** director, Health Research and Studies Center, Los Altos, CA. His study of 16 healthy men and women was presented at an American College of Nutrition symposium on advances in clinical nutrition.

The dietary fiber and tartaric acid that raisins contain help speed food and waste through the digestive system, while also reducing levels of the bile acids that promote tumor growth. The effect is beyond what would be expected from fiber alone. Grapes also contain significant amounts of tartaric acid.

REPORT #75

FOLATE FIGHTS COLORECTAL CANCER

Source: **Paul Terry, PhD, MPH,** department of epidemiology and social medicine, Albert Einstein College of Medicine, Bronx, NY.

Folate is found naturally in asparagus, sunflower seeds, green, leafy vegetables and whole grains. Synthetic folate—folic acid—is often added to breads and cereals. But it is hard to eat enough to get the daily dose of folate that is recommended for cancer protection (at least 400 micrograms), so some people may need a folic-acid supplement. Consult your doctor.

■

REPORT #76
VITAMINS AND COLON POLYPS

Source: **Richard Whelan, MD,** associate professor of surgery and director of colon and rectal surgery, Columbia University College of Physicians and Surgeons, New York City. His four-year study of more than 1,100 patients was published in *Diseases of the Colon & Rectum,* American Society of Colon and Rectal Surgeons, 85 W. Algonquin Rd., Arlington Heights, IL 60005.

Multivitamins and calcium supplements fight precancerous polyps. The use of vitamins and calcium also makes it less likely that colorectal polyps will return in patients who have already had them removed. Nearly all cases of colon and rectal cancer start as benign polyps.

■

REPORT #77
CALCIUM HELPS PREVENT COLON CANCER

Source: **Barbara Levine, PhD, RD,** codirector of the Human Nutrition Program at The Rockefeller University in New York City. She is also director of the Nutrition Information Center and founding director of the Calcium Information Center, both at Weill Medical College of Cornell University–NewYork-Presbyterian Hospital in New York City.

There's overwhelming evidence that adequate levels of dietary calcium can help lower the risk for colon cancer.

Recently, researchers at the Harvard School of Public Health examined the calcium intake and the incidence of colon cancer among more than 130,000 Americans. Those who consumed 1,250 milligrams (mg) or more of calcium a day had a 65% lower risk for colon cancer than those who consumed 500 mg or less.

■

REPORT #78

PANCREATIC CANCER BREAKTHROUGH!

Source: Johns Hopkins School of Medicine, Baltimore, MD.

A new cancer vaccine causes the immune system to destroy pancreatic cancer cells that remain after surgery. In a preliminary study, the vaccine—combined with radiation and chemotherapy—boosted one-year survival rates to 88% from 63% for patients who did not get the vaccine.

REPORT #79

WHAT YOUR DOCTOR ISN'T TELLING YOU: HOW TO PREVENT CANCER

Source: **Richard S. Rivlin, MD,** professor of medicine at Weill Medical College of Cornell University–NewYork-Presbyterian Hospital and director, Anne Fisher Nutrition Center at Strang Cancer Prevention Center, both in New York City. He is also a consultant at Memorial Sloan-Kettering Cancer Center in New York City.

Cancer claims the lives of 1,500 Americans each day. But up to two-thirds of these malignancies could be prevented.

Millions of Americans have taken cancer prevention to heart and made lifestyle changes—eating a nutritious diet, maintaining a healthful weight and not smoking. Now, the latest cancer research has identified other important prevention strategies that most people don't take seriously enough.

Key mistakes…

1. *Inhaling secondhand smoke.* Each year, tobacco use causes approximately 180,000 cancer deaths. Millions of Americans have quit smoking, but most people underestimate the risk of even occasional exposure to secondhand smoke.

The Environmental Protection Agency (EPA) estimates that secondhand smoke causes approximately 3,000 cases of lung cancer in the US annually. If you live with someone who smokes, your risk of dying from lung cancer is 30% higher than if you live in a smoke-free environment.

SELF-DEFENSE: Avoid secondhand smoke by asking guests to smoke outside, for example, or staying away from groups of smokers outside office buildings. This will immediately reduce your risk for cancers of the lung, throat, bladder, kidney, pancreas and mouth.

BONUS: A recent study in the *British Medical Journal* reported that hospital admissions for heart attacks dropped by 60% in Helena, Montana, when the city adopted a smoke-free policy. As little as 30 minutes of exposure to secondhand smoke is hazardous to people with heart or lung conditions.

2. Not getting annual skin exams. There are about one million cases of nonmelanoma skin cancer diagnosed annually in the US—plus more than 54,000 Americans are diagnosed with melanoma, the deadliest skin cancer. Melanoma is 15 to 20 times more common now than it was 50 years ago, in part, because of depletion of the ozone layer.

Skin cancer is among the most preventable and easily treated of all cancers, yet few doctors perform full skin exams during routine checkups. Insist on it. The vast majority of melanomas can be cured if they're detected and treated at an early stage.

SELF-DEFENSE: At least once a year, ask your primary-care physician or dermatologist to check your entire body for any changes in the size or color of moles or other darkly pigmented areas and/or new growths. Make sure your doctor examines areas that are often missed, such as the scalp, soles of the feet and genitals.

SMART IDEA: Ask your doctor to take pictures of suspicious spots that should be watched. The pictures will provide a baseline comparison for future checkups.

3. Settling for sigmoidoscopy. Colon cancer is also among the most treatable of cancers when it's detected early, yet nearly 48,000 Americans die from it needlessly each year.

Unfortunately, many doctors continue to recommend flexible sigmoidoscopy as the only necessary procedure. This test—in which a lighted, hollow tube is inserted through the rectum—views only the lower half of the colon. Cancers or precancerous polyps present in the upper half of the colon are missed entirely by the procedure.

Colonoscopy is a better choice because it views the entire colon. A study that compared the two tests found that nearly half of 128 patients with advanced cancers or adenomas (abnormal growths that can develop into cancer) had them in the upper colon only—the area not examined by sigmoidoscopy.

SELF-DEFENSE: Get a colonoscopy every 10 years, starting at age 50. Patients with risk factors (a family history of colon cancer or a diagnosis of inflammatory bowel disease) may be advised to start getting the test as early as age 35 or 40.

4. *Cutting good dietary fat.* Most Americans have reduced their intake of dietary fat, both for weight control and disease prevention. Studies show that a low-fat diet reduces the risk for a variety of cancers, including malignancies of the colon and prostate.

The saturated fat from animal sources, such as butter and red meat, does appear to elevate cancer risk. But the monounsaturated fats in many nuts, as well as in olive and canola oils, and the omega-3 fatty acids in such cold-water fish as salmon and tuna appear to have anticancer effects. They inhibit the body's production of certain inflammatory *prostaglandins,* natural chemicals that can damage cells and initiate changes that lead to cancer.

A study of more than 6,000 Swedish male twins, recently published in the medical journal *The Lancet,* found that men who did not eat fish were two to three times more likely to get prostate cancer than those who ate fish several times a week. Women who consume large amounts of olive oil may reduce their risk for ovarian cancer by 30%. There's also evidence that olive oil, as well as canola oil, lowers breast cancer risk.

SELF-DEFENSE: Limit all dietary fat to 30% or less of total daily calories...use olive or canola oil to replace butter or vegetable oils (which contain less-healthful polyunsaturated fat)...and substitute several weekly servings of fish for red meat or other foods that are high in saturated fat.

5. *Drinking too much alcohol.* Although it's true that death rates from cardiovascular disease are lower among men and women who drink moderately than among nondrinkers, the benefits are lost with excessive drinking. In fact, the death rates from cancers of the mouth, esophagus, larynx and liver in men and women who consume at least four drinks daily are three to seven times higher than among nondrinkers. Women who drink more than one drink a day are at increased risk for breast cancer.

SELF-DEFENSE: Men should consume no more than two drinks daily—women, no more than one. If you have a family history or another risk factor for breast cancer, it's probably best to forgo a daily drink.

6. Getting "safe" tans. Most Americans know that excessive sun exposure increases the risk for skin cancer, but some still believe that tanning beds are a safe alternative. Not true. People who use tanning beds are 2.5 times more likely to develop squamous cell carcinoma (in the main structural cells of the epidermis) and 1.5 times more likely to get basal cell carcinoma (in the cells at the lowest layer of the epidermis) than those who don't use them. Some tanning salon sessions expose the body to the same amount of harmful ultraviolet A (UVA) radiation as an entire day at the beach.

SELF-DEFENSE: If you still want a tan, try self-tanners, such as those made by Neutrogena or Coppertone, which are sold in most drugstores.

■

REPORT #80

POWERFUL HERBAL MEDICINES PEOPLE RARELY HEAR ABOUT

Source: **James A. Duke, PhD,** leading authority on medicinal plants and former chief, US Department of Agriculture Plant Laboratory, Beltsville, MD. He is author of *Dr. Duke's Essential Herbs: 13 Vital Herbs You Need to Disease-Proof Your Body, Boost Your Energy, and Lengthen Your Life.* Rodale.

Many health consumers are familiar with the top-selling herbal medicines—ginkgo biloba...St. John's wort...and echinacea. There are more than 10,000 medicinal herbs available, which are used to treat a variety of ailments, including flu, varicose veins, the bone-thinning condition known as osteoporosis and hemorrhoids.

Some herbs can work just as well as conventional drugs. Herbs often have fewer side effects, and they usually cost less, too.

ASTRAGALUS (*STRAGALUS MEMBRANACEOUS*)...

This herb has been used for centuries in traditional Chinese medicine in tea or soup, typically in root form.

Also called *huang qi* (pronounced "wahng chee"), astragalus is typically used to bolster the immune system to help the body fight off colds, influenza and harmful bacteria.

TYPICAL DAILY DOSAGE: At the first sign of cold or flu symptoms, prepare a tea of one teaspoon of liquid extract or one-half teaspoon of tincture in one cup of hot water, steeped and drained. Or you can use 2 grams (g) of the root.

CAUTION: Certain species of astragalus are toxic. Do not try to pick and use this herb on your own. Purchase it from a reliable source.

BUTCHER'S BROOM (*RUSCUS ACULEATUS*)...

This herb is often used in Europe for relief from varicose veins and hemorrhoids.

TYPICAL DAILY DOSAGE: Take one 300-milligram (mg) tablet...or 7 to 11 mg of total *ruscogenin*, the active ingredient.

CELERY SEED (*APIUM GRAVEOLENS*)...

The anti-inflammatory properties of celery seed help to ease arthritis and gout symptoms and lower blood pressure.

If you can eat celery without problems, you're unlikely to experience any side effects.

CAUTION: See your doctor before using celery seed for hypertension. It may augment the action of prescription antihypertensives.

TYPICAL DAILY DOSAGE: Take two 500-mg capsules of standardized extract or one-half teaspoon of tincture before meals. For seeds, one tablespoon of seeds in one cup of hot water or added as a spice to soups.

ELDERBERRY (*SAMBUCUS NIGRA*)...

This herb fights viral illnesses, including flu, cold and herpes.

In one study that was conducted during an outbreak of flu in Israel, 90% of people who took a standardized elderberry extract were better within three days.

TYPICAL DAILY DOSAGE: At the onset of flu, cold or herpes, one-half teaspoon of liquid elder flower extract before meals or two to three cups of elder flower tea (two teaspoons of dried elder flowers in one cup of hot water, steeped and drained).

FENUGREEK (*TRIGONELLA FOENUM-GRAECUM*)...

This herb is used to treat diabetes, diarrhea and constipation.

In studies conducted in India, fenugreek was shown to contain five compounds that cause significantly reduced blood sugar levels in people with type 1 or type 2 diabetes.

Fenugreek contains *mucilage*. This soluble fiber absorbs water and provides relief from diarrhea and constipation.

Mucilage also enhances the herb's ability to lower blood sugar levels and may reduce cholesterol and triglyceride levels.

CAUTION: Do not take fenugreek *instead of* prescription diabetes drugs. See your doctor if you want to try this herb to treat diabetes.

TYPICAL DAILY DOSAGE: 620 mg of standardized extract taken before meals, or one cup of fenugreek tea (one tablespoon of mashed seeds steeped in one cup of hot water).

KUDZU (*PUERARIA MONTANA*)...

This herb may help prevent osteoporosis and reduce cravings for alcohol.

Kudzu contains *genistein* and *daidzein*—phytoestrogens that protect against bone loss.

TYPICAL DAILY DOSAGE: Take three 100-mg capsules.

PUMPKIN SEED (*CUCURBITA PEPO*)...

In parts of Europe, pumpkin seeds are the standard treatment for benign prostate enlargement. The seeds are rich in zinc, selenium and other minerals that have been shown to reduce prostate cancer risk.

TYPICAL DAILY DOSAGE: Eat one-quarter cup of the seeds.

USING HERBS SAFELY...

Plant medicines can sometimes intensify or block the effects of prescription drugs. Consult your doctor before taking any herb—especially if you are pregnant, nursing or take prescription medications.

If you're scheduled for surgery, tell your doctor about all the herbs you take...and stop taking them three weeks prior to the procedure. Some herbs reduce—or increase—blood pressure or diminish the effects of anesthesia.

The active ingredients in herbal medicines can vary, depending on the manufacturer. Choose "standardized" brands. These indicate the amount of the active ingredient—and give recommended dosages. You can buy them at health-food stores.

Also, tell your pharmacist about any herbs you are taking, so he/she can monitor possible interactions with prescription drugs.

To find a physician familiar with herbal treatments, contact the American Association of Naturopathic Physicians at 866-538-2267 or *www.naturopathic.org*.

■

REPORT #81

IMPORTANT THERAPIES THAT ARE TOO OFTEN OVERLOOKED

Source: **Kenneth R. Pelletier, MD,** clinical professor of medicine, University of Arizona School of Medicine, Tucson. He is author of *The Best Alternative Medicine: What Works? What Does Not?* Fireside.

Even conservative, traditional doctors have started offering alternative therapies to their patients. They may recommend acupuncture to relieve pain and St. John's wort to curb mild depression.

But there are many effective alternative therapies that remain underused...

BLACK COHOSH...

In Germany, a black cohosh extract called *Remifemin* is frequently prescribed as an alternative to *hormone replacement therapy* (HRT). Preliminary evidence suggests that black cohosh is effective at relieving premenstrual discomfort, menstrual pain and menopausal ailments.

This is good news given the recent evidence linking HRT to increased risk for breast cancer, heart attack, stroke and blood clots.

Any menopausal or postmenopausal woman should ask her doctor about taking black cohosh supplements. They're sold at health-food stores.

CAUTION: Do not take black cohosh for any longer than six months, since no studies have established whether sustained use of this herb is safe.

GUGGUL...

Guggul, an extract from the *mukul myrrh* tree, which is native to India, is used in that country to lower cholesterol. Evidence is mounting that it is effective—and safe. In an Indian study, 40 patients with high cholesterol who took a 25-milligram (mg) supplement of guggul three times a day for 16 weeks cut their total cholesterol an average of 21%. Levels of HDL ("good") cholesterol rose by 35%.

IF YOU HAVE HIGH CHOLESTEROL: Ask your doctor about taking guggul supplements.

MENTAL IMAGERY...

Mental imagery begins with the patient entering a state of deep relaxation similar to that obtained via hypnosis. The physician or hypnotherapist then leads the patient through images in which treatments, recovery and desired outcomes are envisioned.

Mental imagery is of proven effectiveness against chronic pain and anxiety. It has also been used successfully to lower blood pressure and heart rate in heart patients and to improve cancer patients' production of cancer-killing lymphocytes, neutrophils and T-cells.

Writing down thoughts and feelings can be a powerful form of mental imagery. *The Journal of the American Medical Association* published a study of 112 people with asthma or rheumatoid arthritis who all received standard care. In one group, each patient wrote an essay on three consecutive days, describing his/her reaction to a traumatic experience.

RESULT: Four months later, those in the writing group had markedly improved health.

MIND–BODY RELAXATION...

Meditation, hypnosis, stress management and biofeedback are all effective against anxiety and depression, asthma, high blood pressure, chronic pain and carpal tunnel syndrome.

Patients with heart disease who are treated with stress-management classes and muscle tension biofeedback have fewer fatal heart attacks and require fewer heart operations than do similar patients on a standard aerobic exercise program.

Stress-management lessons focus on teaching better coping methods for stressful situations. Methods include visualization, meditative breathing and other relaxation techniques.

Muscle tension biofeedback involves placing electrodes on the skin to measure muscle tension. The patient learns to reduce tension by monitoring a dial or another feedback device.

Anyone who wants to reduce stress or anxiety can consider these techniques. Contact the National Center for Complementary and Alternative Medicine at the National Institutes of Health at 888-644-6226 or *http://nccam.nih.gov*.

PRAYER...

Some studies suggest that prayer promotes healing—even when the patient is unaware of being prayed for. For example, in a study of 393 heart patients at San Francisco General Hospital, half the patients were prayed for, half were not. Neither patients nor doctors knew who had been prayed for.

After 10 months, the prayed-for group had required less medical care—and had lower mortality—than the group not prayed for.

REIKI...

In this laying-on-of-hands technique, a practitioner sends "healing energy" through his hands into the patient's body. Reiki has proven effective in managing pain and healing wounds.

At the University of Michigan Medical School in Ann Arbor, researchers found that Reiki speeds healing of incisions.

People who have chronic pain or feel they are healing too slowly from a wound might want to try Reiki. Contact the International Center for Reiki Training at 800-332-8112 or *www.reiki.org*.

SOY FOODS...

Soy foods are believed to slow menopause onset and prevent bone loss in menopausal women. Now a study at Stanford University School of Medicine suggests that soy is effective when combined with daily supplements of vitamin D and calcium.

Soy derives its effectiveness from estrogen-like compounds known as *phytoestrogens*. Tofu, tempeh, soy milk, edamame (baby soybeans), soy cheese and miso are all rich in phytoestrogens.

Menopausal and postmenopausal women should ask their doctors about taking soy with calcium and vitamin D supplements.

IMPORTANT: Consult your doctor before taking any herbal supplement. Women who are pregnant or nursing should not take herbs.

■

REPORT #82

STRENGTHEN YOUR BODY'S ABILITY TO HEAL ITSELF

Source: **Leo Galland, MD,** director, Foundation for Integrated Medicine, New York City. He has held faculty positions at the Rockefeller University, New York City, and Albert Einstein College of Medicine, Bronx, NY, and is author of *Power Healing.* Random House.

Unscientific as they were by our modern standards, the ancients can teach us a lot about health.

The Greeks and others focused less on specific diseases than on harmony between the mind and body. Maintaining mind–body balance, they knew, keeps us strong. When it is disrupted, we fall prey to illness.

Today, it's possible to have the best of both worlds—the insights of ancient wisdom bolstered by 21st-century science.

POWER HEALING: The four key aspects of my concept of well-being are *relationships*, *diet*, *environment* and *detoxification*.

Strengthening these four pillars of healing will maintain the balance and harmony that protect against illness. If you're ill, these factors will work together with medical care to help you get better.

RELATIONSHIPS...

In recent decades, evidence has grown that strong relationships are a potent force for maintaining good health.

EXAMPLE: A California study found that marriage, close friendships and membership in church or community organizations lowered the overall death rate, as well as the risk of death from cancer, heart disease and stroke.

Good relationships strengthen your ability to deal with stress. The heart is under less strain and the immune system fights off cancer and other diseases better when you feel supported by friends and loved ones.

Social support makes you feel capable of doing positive things—for both yourself and your health.

The first step in strengthening this pillar of healing is to become aware of its importance. **HERE'S HOW...**

• *Take stock.* How much time and energy do you devote to others? What can you do to nurture more gratifying relationships?

• *Make an effort to help others.* Volunteering (at a soup kitchen, hospital, school, museum) reduces stress and eases health problems. By giving to others, you give to yourself.

DIET AND LIFESTYLE...

It should come as no surprise that what you eat has great impact on your health, and that the standard American diet—high in fats, low in vegetables—is a recipe for serious illness.

You can strengthen this pillar of healing dramatically with one *simple step.* Eliminate—or at least *sharply reduce*—your consumption of the junk foods that make up 30% of the average American's calorie intake.

By avoiding processed foods—whose nutrients have been replaced by sugar, salt and shortening—you reduce the risk of heart disease and high blood pressure.

HEALTHFUL SNACKS: When you snack, choose raw vegetables, nuts and seeds rather than junk food.

Two nutrients deserve special attention...

• *Omega-3 fatty acids* have a positive impact on virtually every aspect of cell function. Their gradual disappearance from modern diets has been linked to diseases ranging from arthritis to depression.

Fish that are rich in omega-3s include salmon, albacore tuna and sardines. Flaxseed (oil and flour) is the best vegetable source.

• *Magnesium* regulates the enzyme reactions that support life in virtually every cell, but two-thirds of Americans don't get enough in their diets. Advancing age depletes the body of this mineral, as does stress. You probably need more magnesium if you suffer from irritability...palpitations... muscle tension or spasms.

Green vegetables (especially broccoli), beans, seeds and nuts are good sources of magnesium.

Lifestyle improvements should include regular physical activity. But you don't need to go to a gym. Just incorporate activity into your daily routine—by walking instead of driving the car, for instance.

ENVIRONMENT...

Chemical and biological pollutants wreak havoc with the body, suppressing the immune system, damaging lungs and raising cancer risk, as well as causing minor health problems. Air pollution and toxic dumps are big culprits, but the risk of exposure is greatest indoors. HERE'S WHAT YOU CAN DO...

• *Don't permit smoking in your home.* Secondhand tobacco smoke increases cancer and heart disease risk and aggravates asthma. Carcinogenic tars cling to curtains and furniture.

• *Leave your shoes at the door.* Pesticides and other toxic wastes come in with you off the street, and are collected by carpets.

• *Fight mold.* It can cause severe allergy symptoms, eczema and asthma, as well as fatigue, joint pain and headache. Some types of mold secrete toxins that suppress the immune system. Use a dehumidifier to keep humidity below 50%...discard moldy food...ventilate your basement and attic.

• *Ventilate your stove, heater and dryer properly.* These appliances produce toxic gases, such as carbon monoxide, nitrogen dioxide and formaldehyde.

HELPFUL: Install a carbon monoxide detector.

COST: $50 to $80.

DETOXIFICATION...

Your body has natural defenses against environmental pollutants as well as toxic substances produced by normal cell processes. The liver breaks these pollutants down, at which point they are excreted by the bowels and kidneys. TO ENHANCE AND SUPPORT YOUR BODY'S DETOXIFICATION EFFORTS...

• *Avoid over-the-counter medications when possible.* Many common drugs impair the liver's ability to break down toxic chemicals. Use natural substitutes.

EXAMPLES: *Acetaminophen* (Tylenol) depletes the body of *glutathione*, a key detoxification chemical that protects against cancer and boosts immune function. If you take Tylenol daily, work with your doctor to remedy the source of pain, rather than just treating the symptom. Avoid alcohol, which further depletes glutathione from the liver.

Cimetidine (Tagamet), *ranitidine* (Zantac) and similar drugs widely taken for heartburn impair liver function. Instead, learn strategies to avoid heartburn altogether—eat small, low-fat meals, at least three to four hours before lying down...take chewable calcium with each meal...avoid alcohol and coffee.

• *Actively boost your body's natural detoxification capability.* Do this by consuming foods that neutralize carcinogens and other chemicals that damage cells.

HELPFUL: *Cruciferous* vegetables (such as broccoli, cabbage, brussels sprouts, cauliflower) and those containing *carotenoids* (such as carrots, sweet potatoes, tomatoes).

The herb milk thistle may also be helpful because it protects and improves the liver's efficiency.

The most toxic environment in your body is the digestive tract. You can help your intestines expel toxins by eating more fiber (from fruits, vegetables and whole grains)...and add fermented foods (such as yogurt) to your diet. This will help maintain the healthy bowel bacteria that break down toxins.

■

REPORT #83

HOW TO AVOID "CATCHING" CANCER

Source: **Julie Parsonnet, MD,** professor of infectious diseases and the George DeForest Barnett professor of medicine at Stanford University School of Medicine, Stanford, CA. She is the editor of *Microbes and Malignancy: Infection as a Cause of Human Cancers.* Oxford University.

People tend to think that cancer is caused only by unhealthful personal habits, such as smoking, or environmental factors, including exposure to asbestos or excessive sunlight.

They don't realize that cancer often is triggered by an *infectious* disease.

THE SHOCKER: At least 25% of malignancies are caused by viruses, bacteria and parasites. After smoking, infection is the leading cause of cancer.

Although millions of Americans are infected with cancer-causing organisms at some time during their lives, most of these people don't develop cancer as a result. There are additional risk factors that work in tandem with infectious microbes to trigger the biological changes that lead to cancer.

THE INFECTION LINK...

Viruses are the main cancer-causing organisms, followed by bacteria and parasites. **PRIMARY WAYS THAT THESE ORGANISMS CAUSE CANCER...**

• *Genetic changes.* Viruses can't replicate on their own. When viruses enter your body, they inject their own genetic material into your cells and take over the cells' inner workings.

Some viral genes, known as *oncogenes*, cause cells to divide much more rapidly than usual. Rapid cell division increases the odds of genetic "mistakes" that can lead to cancer. Viruses also inhibit our body's natural ability to destroy damaged cells, which may otherwise continue to grow and divide in ways that make us more vulnerable to cancer.

• *Chronic inflammation.* Some organisms, such as those that cause stomach and liver cancer, irritate tissues and trigger persistent inflammation. Inflammation causes cells to divide at a faster rate than normal, increasing the likelihood that they will mutate and undergo changes that lead to cancer.

CANCER-CAUSING INFECTIONS...

Numerous cancers are believed to be caused, in part, by infectious organisms. **THE MOST COMMON CANCER-CAUSING INFECTIONS—AND STEPS YOU CAN TAKE TO PROTECT YOURSELF...**

• *Helicobacter pylori.* Between 30% and 40% of Americans are infected with Helicobacter pylori, a screw-shaped bacterium that burrows into the stomach lining and causes chronic inflammation. About 20% of these people will eventually develop ulcers—another 5% will develop stomach cancer.

Infection with H. pylori is a very strong risk factor for cancer, presumably because the bacterium causes inflammation and cell proliferation. More than 80% of stomach cancer cases are caused by H. pylori. Infection with this bacterium increases your risk of developing stomach cancer by at least eightfold.

SELF-DEFENSE: Ulcer patients are routinely tested for H. pylori and treated with antibiotics if infection is present. Once the bacterium is eliminated, the risk for ulcers drops significantly.

It is not yet known if treating bacteria will help prevent stomach cancer. Patients with a family history of stomach cancer should talk to their doctors about getting tested for H. pylori.

ALSO HELPFUL: Eat a nutritious diet that is rich in fruits and vegetables and low in salt and food preservatives known as nitrates. Such a diet may reduce cancer risk.

• *Epstein-Barr virus.* The Epstein-Barr virus (EBV) causes infectious mononucleosis, which leads to extreme fatigue and other flu-like symptoms. EBV is found in the tumors of a significant number of patients with Hodgkin's disease (a form of lymphoma that strikes most often between the ages of 15 to 35 and after age 55).

The risk that an individual patient who has had mononucleosis will go on to develop Hodgkin's disease—or non-Hodgkin's lymphoma, which also is associated with the EBV virus—is still very low.

The main risk for non-Hodgkin's lymphoma appears to be in patients who have severely compromised immune systems—for example, those who have undergone transplant surgery and/or are taking immune-suppressing drugs.

SELF-DEFENSE: Transmission of EBV is impossible to prevent because many healthy people can carry and spread the virus for life.

People who receive transplants and immune-suppressing drugs should ask their doctors about symptoms of EBV-related malignancies. Decreasing immunosuppression can often reverse lymphoma when caught early.

• *Hepatitis B.* The hepatitis B virus (HBV) is spread by contact with body fluids of an infected person, including blood, saliva, vaginal secretions and semen.

AT GREATEST RISK: People who have sex with infected partners...and drug users who share needles.

Most cases of HBV are *acute*, lasting six months or less. This form of hepatitis is not linked to cancer. However, the *chronic* form of HBV, which is almost always acquired in childhood and lasts for more than six months, greatly increases the risk for cirrhosis (destruction of normal liver tissue) as well as liver cancer.

SELF-DEFENSE: All newborns are now given the HBV vaccine. It's also recommended for children ages 18 years or younger who weren't previously vaccinated.

Adults don't require the vaccine for cancer prevention— but it is recommended for those in high-risk groups because it can reduce the risk for long-term liver disease.

AMONG THOSE WHO SHOULD GET THE HBV VACCINE: Healthcare workers...those who are sexually active with people who may have HBV and/or have household contact with them... and dialysis patients.

• *Hepatitis C.* Most people with the hepatitis C virus (HCV) were infected by tainted blood transfusions prior to 1992, when blood-screening tests first became available. HCV also can be transmitted by having sex with someone who is infected ...sharing contaminated hypodermic needles...and receiving nonsterile tattoo or body-piercing procedures.

About 5% of patients with HCV will develop liver cancer. A much higher percentage will develop cirrhosis or other chronic liver diseases—usually decades after the initial exposure.

SELF-DEFENSE: In addition to the high-risk practices mentioned above, do not share razors, toothbrushes or nail clippers in households with an HCV-infected person.

Patients who received a blood transfusion prior to 1992, or who engage in high-risk practices, should be tested for HCV.

Treatment depends on the type and extent of the HCV infection. For example, a combination of *interferon* (such as PEG-INTRON) and an antiviral drug called *ribavirin* (Rebetol) can eliminate infection in 50% to 80% of cases.

• *Human papilloma virus.* A majority of sexually active American women will be exposed to one of the many strains of human papilloma virus (HPV) at some time during their lives. HPV is a sexually transmitted infection that may cause no symptoms itself but increases the risk for cervical cancer.

Fortunately, only a small percentage of women with HPV go on to develop cervical cancer. There also are relatively harmless forms of HPV, such as those that cause genital warts—these do *not* increase cancer risk.

An HPV vaccine was recently approved by the US Food and Drug Administration (FDA) and appears to be extremely effective.

The use of condoms and other safe-sex practices aren't very effective at preventing the spread of HPV. That's because condoms may not cover enough of the penis to prevent exposure. The virus also can be transmitted by hand-to-genital contact.

SELF-DEFENSE: Women should get regular Pap tests to look for precancerous changes in the cervix. The American Cancer Society recommends an HPV test in addition to a Pap smear for women ages 30 and older. The cure rate for cervical cancer is about 90% when it's detected at an early stage.

■

REPORT #84

MAGNIFY YOUR MIND POWER

Source: **Arthur Winter, MD,** assistant professor of neurosurgery at New Jersey Medical College and director of New Jersey Neurological Institute, both in Livingston. He is coauthor of *Brain Workout* (ASJA Press) and *Build Your Brain Power* (St. Martin's Press).

What you eat has a direct effect on your brain. Some foods improve your ability to concentrate. Others aid memory and facilitate the ability to solve problems. Still others generate hormones that stabilize mood and enhance concentration. **HERE ARE SOME IMPORTANT BRAIN NUTRIENTS AND THE FOODS THAT CONTAIN THEM...**

CHOLINE...

Choline is a fatlike substance related to the B vitamins. It is converted in the brain into *acetylcholine*, a neurotransmitter linked to memory and cognitive function. You should make every effort to get adequate choline as you age because the level of the enzyme needed to produce it, *N-acetyltransferase*, declines as we age. People with Alzheimer's disease have been found to have significantly reduced levels of acetylcholine.

In laboratory studies, animals given choline-enhanced diets for several months were able to form new long-term memories more efficiently than animals on standard diets. It's not clear if supplemental choline is beneficial to humans, but adequate dietary amounts are essential for normal brain function and may play a role in preserving brain function in people with Alzheimer's and other neurological diseases.

RECOMMENDED: One or more servings daily of high-choline foods—egg yolks, dairy, soy, beef, liver, wheat germ, oatmeal, brown rice, peanuts and fish.

VITAMIN B-12...

Vitamin B-12 is used to produce *myelin*, which is the sheathing on nerve cells. A deficiency can cause impaired transmission of nerve signals as well as declines in memory and other cognitive functions.

NEW FINDING: B-12 inhibits the activity of *monoamine oxidase* (MAO), an enzyme that breaks down brain chemicals. Alzheimer's patients given supplemental B-12 have improved memory and communication skills.

RECOMMENDED: Two to three servings weekly of B-12-rich liver, red meat, eggs or dairy. Everyone should take a daily multivitamin and mineral supplement for insurance. People who follow a strict vegan diet (no animal foods) should also supplement with six micrograms (mcg) of B-12 daily.

Ask your doctor to check your blood level of vitamin B-12 if you're experiencing memory problems. More than 20% of older adults have low levels of vitamin B-12 because they lack *intrinsic factor*, a stomach protein required for B-12 absorption. Deficiencies of B-12 are thought to account for 10% of non-Alzheimer's memory loss cases. People with inadequate intrinsic factor require monthly intramuscular B-12 injections.

AMINO ACIDS...

The brain is almost completely regulated by amino acids, the 20 different building blocks of protein. Nine of these—the essential amino acids—can be derived from diet only. People who eat a well-balanced diet almost always get adequate amino acids. Supplemental amounts may offer additional protection, but this hasn't been established. Promising amino acids include *tyrosine* (involved in alertness), *phenylalanine* (linked to memory) and *methionine* (involved in motivation and focus).

RECOMMENDED: 45 grams (g) to 75 g of dietary protein daily —about three servings. Protein from animal foods, such as beef, chicken, fish and dairy, are complete and contain all of the necessary amino acids. Vegetable proteins (with the exception of soy) don't contain all of the essential amino acids. Vegetarians should eat a variety of high-protein foods daily, such as combining nuts with legumes, to achieve the proper balance.

FOLIC ACID...

Another B vitamin, folic acid, appears to affect brain function. One study found that older adults with dementia or other mental disorders were three times more likely than normal adults to have low levels of folic acid. Deficiencies of folic acid have been linked with declines in memory and abstract thinking ability.

RECOMMENDED: Along with a multivitamin, eat two servings daily of foods high in folic acid—asparagus, leafy green vegetables, lentils, wheat, fortified cereals, meat and broccoli.

As little as 200 mcg of folic acid (the amount in three-quarters of a cup of cooked spinach) has been shown to improve mood and relieve depression and fatigue in healthy older people.

VITAMIN C...

The brain and adrenal glands are the body's main repositories of vitamin C. Because the adrenal glands produce stress-related hormones, it is suspected that vitamin C may play a role in modulating physical and emotional stress.

Stress elevates levels of the hormone *cortisol*, which can eventually damage cells in the hippocampus, the part of the brain involved in memory. Vitamin C is a powerful antioxidant that can minimize physical stress to brain tissue caused by such factors as smoking, alcohol consumption and air pollution.

Vitamin C also assists in the production of neurotransmitters and participates in the processing of glucose, the brain's primary fuel. One study found that people with low blood levels of vitamin C scored lower on memory tests than those with normal levels.

RECOMMENDED: Two daily servings of vitamin C–rich foods—which include citrus fruits and juices, tomatoes, strawberries and potatoes. Most Americans should get at least 100 milligrams (mg) of vitamin C daily—more if you smoke or drink alcohol. One orange has about 70 mg.

COMPLEX CARBOHYDRATES...

The brain depends almost entirely on glucose—derived from the breakdown of carbohydrates—for energy. Glucose provides the energy that the brain needs for concentration and other cognitive functions, and it has been shown to enhance memory and improve performance on standardized tests.

CAUTION: A diet high in simple sugars (from pastries, soft drinks, candy, etc.) triggers hormonal changes that cause drops in blood glucose, which increases fatigue and impairs memory and concentration. Stroke patients with excessive blood sugar suffer more nerve and brain damage than those with lower levels.

RECOMMENDED: Avoid sugar. Get glucose from complex carbohydrates, such as whole grains, legumes, fruits and vegetables. About half of your daily caloric intake should come from these foods.

THE TOP 10...

The best foods for your brain include...
- *Low-fat milk or yogurt*
- *Eggs*
- *Lean meats, such as flank steak*
- *Poultry*
- *Spinach and other leafy greens*
- *Whole-wheat bread*
- *Oranges*
- *Black beans and other legumes*
- *Enriched brown rice*
- *Salmon*

REPORT #85

PUT THE BRAKES ON PARKINSON'S

Source: **Stanley Fahn, MD,** H. Houston Merritt professor of neurology and director, Center for Parkinson's Disease and Other Movement Disorders at Columbia University in New York City. He is also scientific director of the Parkinson's Disease Foundation, past president of the American Academy of Neurology and founder of the Movement Disorder Society.

Parkinson's disease, the second most common degenerative brain disease (after Alzheimer's), affects 1 million Americans and typically begins between ages 50 and 79. Characterized by tremor, slowness of movement, stiffness of the limbs and trunk, difficulty walking and lack of facial expression, the disease has no known cause. There is no preventive or cure for Parkinson's disease, but research is now making advances in both areas.

LATEST DEVELOPMENT: For the first time ever, renowned neuroscientists, doctors and other health-care workers joined Parkinson's patients and their family members at the recent World Parkinson Congress in Washington, DC, to discuss innovative therapies that show promise in controlling symptoms as well as restoring motor function.

HOW PARKINSON'S DEVELOPS...

Parkinson's disease occurs when nerve cells (neurons) that control movement start to die off for unknown reasons. The result is a shortage of the brain-signaling chemical *dopamine,* which triggers the muscles that allow fluid body movements, such as lifting an arm or walking.

The decline in dopamine levels leads to tremor, incoordination, slowed, reduced movement and other Parkinson's symptoms.

Research reported at the congress...

COENZYME Q10...

NEW FINDING: A small National Institutes of Health (NIH)–funded trial of coenzyme Q10 (a natural nutrient, also known as CoQ10, that is present in all human cells) found that taking

1,200 milligrams (mg) daily may slow disease progression in patients with early-stage Parkinson's.

More study is needed to confirm that CoQ10 does indeed slow the progression of the disease. Because the dosage of CoQ10 that was studied is only mildly effective, additional research also is needed to determine whether a higher dose (2,400 mg of CoQ10 daily) works better.

IMPLICATION: Parkinson's patients who are eager to try all possible therapies should ask their doctors about taking 1,200 mg daily of CoQ10. No side effects have been shown at this dosage.

DOPAMINE AGONISTS...

Levodopa, also known as *L-dopa* (Larodopa), is the gold standard in treating Parkinson's. But many patients taking levodopa eventually develop uncontrolled flailing movements—a condition called *dyskinesia*—and motor fluctuations, in which medication levels in the brain drop and Parkinson's symptoms return.

Some doctors prefer to hold off prescribing levodopa in favor of a drug known as a *dopamine agonist*, which mimics the effects of dopamine in the brain and causes neurons to react as though sufficient amounts of dopamine were present. Dopamine agonists reduce Parkinson's-related disabilities—and work even better when combined with levodopa.

Dopamine agonists approved by the FDA are *bromocriptine* (Parlodel), *pergolide* (Permax), *pramipexole* (Mirapex), *ropinirole* (Requip) and *apomorphine* (Apokyn). Rotigotine, the only dopamine agonist offered in patch form, is available in Europe. The FDA could approve the drug as early as 2007. The patch may be desirable for patients who have trouble swallowing or want the convenience of using a patch once a day.

NEW FINDING: In a two-year study of 186 early-stage Parkinson's patients, brain scans of those taking ropinirole or levodopa suggest that dopamine agonists may slow the decline of Parkinson's disease. Levodopa was found to worsen the disease, although patients' symptoms improved.

IMPLICATION: Because medications may interfere with brain scan results, more study is needed to confirm these findings. Ropinirole should be considered as treatment. Among the most likely candidates are younger patients who experience motor fluctuations and dyskinesia from levodopa.

IMPORTANT: Ropinirole has been shown to cause side effects, such as sleepiness, nausea, hallucinations and, in rare cases, odd behavior, such as compulsive shopping and gambling.

MINOCYCLINE AND CREATINE...

NEW FINDING: In an NIH-sponsored clinical trial, 200 Parkinson's patients who did not yet require medication were randomly assigned to receive 200 mg daily of the antibiotic *minocycline*, 10 grams (g) daily of *creatine* (a nutritional supplement used to increase lean body mass and strength) or a placebo for 12 months.

Minocycline was studied due to its anti-inflammatory effects. Inflammation has been detected in the brains of Parkinson's patients. Creatine is an energy booster, and decreased energy utilization is a problem in Parkinson's disease. Minocycline and creatine were found to be potentially beneficial.

IMPLICATION: More study is needed before minocycline or creatine can be prescribed as a treatment for Parkinson's disease.

DEEP BRAIN STIMULATION...

NEW FINDING: An advanced surgical technique known as deep brain stimulation (DBS) has been shown to provide significant benefit to moderate and advanced Parkinson's patients for up to four years after the onset of treatment.

With DBS, a surgeon implants an electrode inside the brain to stimulate specific brain sites that control movement. The electrode is connected to a palm-sized pacemaker that is implanted beneath the skin just below the clavicle. By stimulating key parts of the brain, the pacemaker helps alleviate motor symptoms, such as tremor.

Serious complications from DBS, such as stroke, occur in fewer than 2% of patients. More common side effects include speech impairment, personality and/or mood change, depression and a decline in cognitive function in older patients.

IMPLICATION: DBS is especially helpful for people who respond to levodopa but suffer from dyskinesia and wearing off of the drug. DBS is covered by Medicare and many other forms of health insurance.

TYPICAL COST: $30,000 to $60,000.

REPORT #86

MAGNIFY YOUR MEMORY

Source: **Adriane Fugh-Berman, MD**, a Washington, DC–based medical researcher who specializes in women's health and alternative medicine. She is author of *Alternative Medicine: What Works.* Lippincott Williams & Wilkins.

Do you—or does someone you love—keep losing keys, forgetting names or having other memory lapses? If so, you may be worried that the culprit is Alzheimer's disease or another incurable form of dementia. While it's a good idea to consult a doctor, the odds are that it is simple forgetfulness—which can be treated.

In some cases, memory problems—especially those associated with aging—stem simply from a lack of mental activity. If your job isn't particularly stimulating—or if you're retired—you might consider keeping a journal, joining a book discussion group, playing chess or Scrabble, doing crossword puzzles, etc.

Physical exercise is also a memory-enhancer. Aerobic exercise boosts circulation throughout the body—and that includes the brain.

Another way to ensure adequate blood flow to the brain is to eat a low-fat diet. The arteries that feed the brain are tiny to begin with, and any narrowing that occurs as a result of eating a fatty or cholesterol-rich diet drastically reduces oxygen flow. Blood flow problems can lead to tiny strokes, which are now believed to be the cause of much age-related memory loss.

These strokes—which generally produce no obvious symptoms—are typically caused by chronic high blood pressure and/or high cholesterol. So be sure your blood pressure and cholesterol are under control.

While there's no magic memory pill, the following supplements are safe...and beneficial for many people. They can be taken individually or in combination. For absolute safety, use them under a doctor's supervision.

• *Antioxidants.* Vitamins C and E and the mineral selenium all may help prevent memory loss. I usually tell my patients to take 400 international units (IU) of vitamin E a day,* along

*Consult your doctor for the amount that is appropriate for you.

with 1,000 milligrams (mg) of vitamin C and 100 micrograms (mcg) of selenium. It's also a good idea to eat lots of fruits and vegetables. They contain lots of other antioxidants.

• *Phosphatidylserine.* This fatty substance was found to be helpful in preventing further deterioration in people with memory problems. In some cases, memory *improved* after several months of phosphatidylserine therapy. I usually recommend 200 to 300 mg per day. Be patient—it may take three months before you notice any improvement.

Some alternative practitioners recommend a related substance called *choline* (or *lecithin,* which contains 10% to 20% choline). Neither choline nor lecithin looks anywhere near as good as phosphatidylserine, and they can cause unpleasant side effects.

• *L-acetyl carnitine.* This form of the amino acid carnitine plays a key role in energy production in the body. It seems to help both Alzheimer's patients and those with mild mental deterioration. The usual dose is 500 mg to 1,000 mg three times a day.

• *Ginkgo biloba.* Like vitamin E, ginkgo helps thin the blood, boosting circulation inside even the tiniest capillaries—including those that feed the brain. Ginkgo also acts as an antioxidant, protecting the brain against attack by free radicals.

Ginkgo has been found to be effective in slowing the progression of Alzheimer's disease.

■

REPORT #87

LEMON BALM HELPS RECALL

Source: **David Kennedy, PhD,** professor of psychobiology and psychology at Northumbria University, Newcastle upon Tyne, England.

In one study, the participants who took standardized word- and picture-recall tests scored significantly better several hours after taking a 1,600-milligram (mg) capsule of dried lemon balm leaf than when they were given a placebo.

THEORY: The herb binds to brain chemical receptors, enhancing their ability to send and receive information.

what to do: Add three teaspoons (or three tea bags) of dried lemon balm to two cups of boiling water. Steep for five minutes and then strain. Drink daily. Or take a 1,600-mg supplement daily.

■

REPORT #88

INCONTINENCE CURED

Source: **Jonathan M. Vapnek, MD,** urologist, associate clinical professor of urology and director of neurourology at Mount Sinai School of Medicine in New York City. He is a member of the American Urological Association and has been named by *New York* magazine as one of New York City's best urologists.

For the estimated 13 million Americans with urinary incontinence, poor bladder control can severely disrupt daily life. Some people don't always make it to the bathroom in time or they can't hold it in when they cough or sneeze. Some even curtail social activities because they don't have reliable bladder control.

Yet the majority of people with this condition never see a doctor—either because they're too embarrassed to discuss it or because they assume that it's a normal part of getting older.

Not true. About 80% of patients can regain nearly normal bladder control with lifestyle changes or, if necessary, medication or surgery.

TYPES OF INCONTINENCE...

As the bladder fills with urine, it eventually sends signals to the brain that tell the person "it's time to go." Before that happens, the bladder walls relax to permit urine to accumulate. This gradual process is what allows most people to wait hours before going to the bathroom. Urinary control also is achieved by a ring of muscle called the urinary sphincter. It contracts to keep urine in, then relaxes to let it out.

Incontinence occurs when a person has a problem with either muscular or nervous system control—or a combination of both. Women are about twice as likely as men to have incontinence, although men who have prostate enlargement or have had prostate surgery have an increased risk of incontinence.

The main types...

• *Stress incontinence* is most common, affecting at least 50% of the women who have urinary incontinence. It occurs when the urinary sphincter isn't strong enough to hold in urine, particularly during activities that cause an increase in abdominal pressure, including laughing, coughing, sneezing and exercise.

Stress incontinence frequently occurs during pregnancy and can persist in women who have had several vaginal births. Large babies and long labors can stretch and weaken the pelvic floor muscles and/or damage some of a woman's bladder nerves. The drop in estrogen that occurs after menopause can weaken the urethra, inhibiting its ability to hold back the flow of urine.

• *Urge incontinence* often is caused by inflammation or irritation of the bladder or urethra—due to infection, urinary stones or, in men, irritation of the prostate gland. This causes frequent (and sudden) urges to urinate. This type of incontinence also may be caused by bowel problems and neurological problems, such as stroke or Parkinson's disease.

• *Overflow incontinence.* Patients with nerve damage (from diabetes, for example) or damage to the bladder may constantly dribble urine because they're unable to empty the bladder completely when they urinate.

Other potential causes of incontinence are an enlarged prostate gland, a tumor in the urinary tract or bladder cancer. The majority of patients have either stress or urge incontinence—or a combination of both, known as mixed incontinence.

DIAGNOSIS...

Most cases and types of incontinence can be diagnosed with a medical history alone. Keep a bladder diary for a week or two before you see your doctor. Write down how often you urinate...when you leak...and if you have trouble emptying your bladder. The answers to these questions usually are sufficient to allow a definitive diagnosis.

Tests may be required to provide additional information.
MOST COMMON...

• *Stress test.* The doctor examines the urethra while the patient coughs or bears down. A leakage of urine indicates that the patient has stress incontinence.

• *Urodynamic testing.* There are a variety of tests that measure pressure in the bladder and how much fluid it can hold.

EXAMPLE: The doctor might insert a catheter into the bladder, inject small amounts of fluid and measure changes in bladder pressure. Sudden increases in bladder pressure and/or spasms could indicate urge incontinence.

Patients may require an ultrasound to check how well the bladder empties. Your doctor also should perform urinalysis to check for blood or signs of infection in the urine.

TREATMENT...

Some forms of incontinence are transitory and will go away when the underlying problem (an infection or inflammation, for example) improves. Most incontinence requires one or more of the following treatments, which can bring about significant improvement for most patients.

• *Behavioral techniques.* These techniques are used to help patients achieve better bladder control and are considered the mainstay of treatment. **EXAMPLES...**

• Bladder training requires patients to avoid going to the bathroom for longer and longer periods. A person might try to wait an extra 10 minutes when he/she has the urge to urinate. The goal is to lengthen the waiting time over a period of days or weeks. With practice, most patients are able to wait several hours. This is for patients with bladder overactivity and frequent urination.

• Timed urination means going to the bathroom at specific intervals—say, once every hour, even if you don't feel as though you have to go. This might be used for frail, elderly people who tend to wet themselves because they can't hold it once the urge hits. The idea is to void before the bladder hits that point of no return.

• Kegel exercises. Patients are advised to tightly squeeze the same muscles that they would use to stop the flow of urine. Contract the muscles for three to five seconds, relax, then repeat again. Do the cycle several times daily, working up to more repetitions each time. Kegels are helpful for men and women and for both stress and urge incontinence cases.

• *Medications.* Antispasmodic drugs reduce bladder contractions that contribute to urge incontinence. These drugs often cause dry mouth as a side effect. They're usually used in combination with behavioral treatments.

• *Surgery.* If behavioral changes and medications don't adequately control incontinence, patients may require surgery.

MAIN APPROACHES...

• Tension-free vaginal tape (TVT) procedure. This is standard for women with stress incontinence. A mesh-like tape is slung under the urethra like a hammock. It compresses the urethra to prevent leaks.

• Bulking injections. Collagen or synthetic bulking agents are injected into tissue surrounding the urethra or urinary sphincter. The extra bulk causes surrounding tissue to tighten the seal of the sphincter. The procedure usually needs to be repeated every six to 18 months because collagen is absorbed by the body over time.

• Sphincter replacement. An artificial, doughnut-shaped device is implanted around the urethra. When patients are ready to urinate, they press a valve that causes the device to deflate and let out urine. This procedure is mainly used for men who have had prostate surgery.

REPORT #89

BEAT BAD BREATH

Source: **Mark A. Stengler, ND,** naturopathic physician in private practice, La Jolla, CA...associate clinical professor at the National College of Naturopathic Medicine, Portland, OR...author of numerous books, including *The Natural Physician's Healing Therapies* and coauthor of *Prescription for Natural Cures* (both from Bottom Line Books)...and author of the *Bottom Line/Natural Healing* newsletter.

About half of Americans have bad breath (*halitosis*). Fortunately, a simple natural approach often is all it takes to eradicate the problem.

Several conditions may contribute to bad breath, including gum disease, degrading silver fillings, chronic dental and/or throat infections and ulcers and other digestive problems. It is important to work with your dentist to determine the cause because bad breath may indicate a bigger problem. **IF YOUR DENTIST CAN'T FIND A PROBLEM, TRY THESE SUGGESTIONS...**

Take one teaspoon of liquid *chlorophyll* (the green pigment in plants) straight or diluted in a glass of water after meals. Chlorophyll (available at most health-food stores) freshens breath immediately and supports detoxification of the digestive tract.

Many people who have bad breath have an overgrowth of bacteria in the mouth, which is typically caused by certain foods, sugar, lack of good bacteria and/or infection. For these cases, I recommend rinsing with *xylitol*, a natural sugar alcohol found in many fruits, berries, vegetables and mushrooms. Xylitol prevents bacteria from adhering to teeth and gums.

I have seen good results with a product called Spry Coolmint Oral Rinse, which should be used twice daily. It is available at many health-food stores and some dentists' offices.

■

REPORT #90

WHAT BACK SURGEONS DON'T WANT YOU TO KNOW

Source: British Medical Journal.

B ritish researchers say there's no clear evidence that spinal fusion surgery for chronic low back pain is better than intensive rehabilitation in relieving discomfort.

What's more, these surgeries may not be as cost-effective as other interventions, they add.

THE STUDY...

The study included 349 people who experienced chronic low back pain, defined as pain lasting more than a year. **PATIENTS WERE DIVIDED INTO TWO GROUPS:** 176 underwent spinal fusion surgery and 173 were enrolled in an intensive rehabilitation program that included daily exercises and cognitive (mental) behavior therapy.

During the two years of the study, 38 of the patients assigned to the rehabilitation group had received surgery as well, compared with seven surgery patients who had received both treatments.

This finding seems to indicate that surgery has a slight advantage over rehabilitation. However, the study authors believe the benefit is still too small, considering the potential risk and financial expense of surgery.

CONCLUSION...

The researchers say there is no clear proof that surgery is better than rehabilitation, and suggest that rehabilitation should routinely be made available to people who have chronic low back pain.

Their cost analysis also found that, on average, surgery is much more expensive per patient than rehabilitation.

However, the researchers caution, this conclusion could change if more patients who receive rehabilitation go on to require back surgery in the future.

The National Institute of Neurological Disorders and Stroke has more information about back pain at *www.ninds.nih.gov*. Click on "Disorders."

REPORT #91

YOGA FOR BEGINNERS

Source: **Alice Christensen,** founder and executive director, American Yoga Association, 513 S. Orange Ave., Sarasota, FL 34236. She is author of *20-Minute Yoga Workouts*. Ballantine.

If you're chronically anxious or simply feel "stressed out," consider giving yoga a try. This 5,000-year-old system of exercise, breathing and meditation is wonderfully effective at clearing the mind and easing muscular tension.

It also fosters a profound sense of self-confidence—a feeling that you can handle whatever comes your way.

BASIC YOGA PROGRAM...

A basic program takes about 20 minutes each day. Some people prefer doing yoga in the morning. Others prefer early evening. Either way is okay. Just make sure you do it at the same time of day—every day.

The only "equipment" you'll need is a quiet room...loose, comfortable clothing...and a blanket, large towel or another pad on which to sit comfortably.*

YOGA BREATHING...

To help focus your attention inward, start with two minutes of "complete breath" exercises.

Sit cross-legged on a firm cushion on the floor, or find another seated position in which your back is straight but also relaxed.

Begin inhaling slowly and deeply through the nose. Relax your belly so that it expands with each incoming breath, and let your chest and rib cage expand. At the very "top" of each inhalation, your shoulders will lift slightly. At this point, exhale by relaxing your shoulders and then your ribs. Then tighten your belly to squeeze the air out. Relax and repeat.

IMPORTANT: When we breathe ordinarily, each inhalation lasts longer than each exhalation. With yoga breathing, inhalation and exhalation should take the same amount of time.

Breathe *in* for a count of five...then *out* for a count of five until you've established a rhythm. Then focus on the sound of your breath.

ARM AND SHOULDER STRETCHES...

These three stretches—each done while standing—loosen the joints and ease muscular tension.

• *Arm roll.* Hold your arms out to the side, elbows straight, hands held up as if stopping traffic. Rotate your arms forward in three large circles, then backward in three large circles. Then do three *small* circles in each direction.

• *Head roll.* With arms at your sides, bend your head forward while relaxing the muscles in the back of your neck. Slowly tilt your head to one side, then back, then to the other side, then to the front.

*For more information on yoga, or to order videos or audiotapes, contact the American Yoga Association at 941-927-4977, *www.americanyogaassociation.org.*

Do this head rotation three times clockwise, then three times counterclockwise.

• *Side stretch.* Keep your feet slightly more than shoulder-width apart, with arms held out to the side. Inhale deeply. Then exhale as you bend to the right. Slide your right hand down your right thigh toward the knee, and bring your left arm overhead. Breathe in, and return to an upright position.

Do the same stretch on your left side. Repeat three times on each side.

SPINE STRETCHES...

These poses are especially beneficial if you work at a desk.

• *Sun pose.* Stand with feet together. As you inhale, raise your arms from the side until they're overhead. Look upward. Exhale as you bend from the waist. Reach as far forward as you comfortably can, and grasp your ankles, calves or knees.

Hold for a moment, then inhale as you return to an upright position, raising arms to the side until they're overhead. Lower arms in a circle as you exhale. Repeat twice.

• *Baby pose.* Sit on your feet. Slowly bend forward until your head approaches the floor. Let your arms rest at your sides with elbows bent. Hold for at least one minute.

• *Corpse pose.* Lie on your back with feet slightly apart and arms at sides, palms up. Close your eyes. Relax your entire body, paying particular attention to the face and stomach. Rest for at least one minute.

YOGA MEDITATION...

Meditation teaches us to *observe*—rather than worry about or act upon—the thoughts that constantly flit through our minds.

This lets us withdraw from the never-ending bombardment of desires, fears, regrets, etc....and find peace by turning our attention solely to the present moment. Start by lying face up on your pad, with arms at sides, palms up. Remain as still as possible.

For the next two minutes or so, focus on each part of your body in turn. Envision each part separately...and relax it.

Start with your forehead, then your eyes, face, neck and shoulders. Move down your body, relaxing each in turn—arms and hands...chest and abdomen...hips, legs and feet...then back up the spine to the neck and head.

Gently bring your attention to your forehead. Silently repeat "om" several times.

Your aim is to think of nothing. If thoughts intrude, don't worry—and don't try to *force* them to stop. Gently return your attention to the experience of silence.

TRAP: The more you fight to *control* your thoughts, the harder your thoughts will resist you. Instead, just observe the thoughts as if they were passing by in the distance.

After meditating for 10 minutes or so, open your eyes. Wiggle your fingers and toes, open and close your fists. Take a deep breath. Stretch your arms and legs. Your yoga session is over.

As you become more skilled at meditation, you should be able to *remember* and *reproduce* the feeling at will—to achieve instant relaxation anytime, anywhere.

REPORT #92

THE AMAZING "VITAMIN K CURE" FOR OSTEOPOROSIS

Source: **Harris H. McIlwain, MD,** chair of the Florida Osteoporosis Board and adjunct professor, University of South Florida College of Public Health in Tampa. He is a board-certified rheumatologist and founder of the Tampa Medical Group. Dr. McIlwain is coauthor, with Debra Fulghum Bruce, PhD, and his daughters Laura McIlwain Cruse, MD, and Kimberly McIlwain Smith, MD, of *Reversing Osteopenia: The Definitive Guide to Recognizing and Treating Early Bone Loss in Women of All Ages.* Henry Holt.

M ost women—as well as men—who are past age 50 know that they are at risk for osteoporosis, the leading cause of bone fractures in older adults. But few older adults realize that they also are at risk for a precursor to osteoporosis known as *osteopenia.*

NEW FINDING: Estimates suggest that half of all women over age 45 and about 30% of men of the same age group have the mild bone loss that characterizes osteopenia.

Painful bone fractures, which are commonly associated with osteoporosis, also can occur in people who have osteopenia. These fractures can cause spinal deformities...hand or wrist disability...and severe hip injury.

SAY GOODBYE TO BONE...

In women and men, new bone is constantly being produced and old bone broken down in a process called *remodeling*.

Until recently, doctors believed that a woman's peak bone-building years began in her childhood and extended to her 20s or 30s.

NEW FINDING: Bone growth slows significantly about 10 years earlier than previously thought.

For women, when estrogen levels decline at menopause, bone loss accelerates greatly. In the first five years after menopause, some women lose up to 25% of bone density.

Typically, men start to lose bone 10 years later than women. Testosterone deficiency and the use of certain steroid medications, such as *prednisone* (Deltasone), are some of the most common causes.

RISK FACTORS...

A sedentary lifestyle, not getting enough bone-building calcium and vitamin D, and low body weight in women (less than 127 pounds) are the main causes of osteopenia.

Other key risk factors...

• *Very low-calorie diets.* Men and women who severely restrict calories—for example, consuming fewer than 1,000 to 1,200 calories daily—may not get enough dietary protein to ensure healthy bone growth.

• *Cola consumption.* Research has shown that drinking more than one 12-ounce cola daily significantly lowers bone density. That may be because cola contains phosphoric acid, which blocks calcium absorption.

• *Smoking.* It doubles the risk for developing osteopenia in both women and men.

EARLY DETECTION...

All menopausal and postmenopausal women as well as women and men of any age with two or more of the risk factors listed above should get a bone-density test.

The most accurate test is dual energy X-ray absorptiometry (DEXA). It is painless and takes only about 10 minutes and exposes patients to less radiation than that used for a chest X ray. It usually costs $100 to $125 and is covered by most insurance plans.

DEXA measures bone mineral density and converts the measurement into a standardized value called a T-score. The result shows how a patient's bone density compares with that of a typical 25-year-old woman. A higher T-score means stronger bones. A normal T-score is above -1.0...osteopenia, -1.0 to -2.5...and full-fledged osteoporosis, less than -2.5. If your results are abnormal, the test should be repeated every one to two years.

MAINTAINING BONE STRENGTH...

Patients can stop further bone loss—or, in some cases, reverse osteopenia—with lifestyle steps...

• *Get adequate calcium.* You've heard it before—but there's no way around the importance of calcium. From age 25 to menopause, women need 1,200 milligrams (mg) daily, and 1,500 mg daily thereafter. Men need 1,000 mg daily from age 30 to 65, and 1,500 mg daily thereafter.

Dairy foods, including milk, have long been the most popular sources of calcium. An eight-ounce glass of milk provides about 300 mg—but only 25% to 30% of the mineral is actually absorbed.

WHAT MOST PEOPLE DON'T KNOW: Juice can be a better calcium source than milk. An eight-ounce glass of calcium-fortified orange juice contains 350 mg (36% absorption).

Absorption rates are useful to know, so you can choose your calcium sources wisely. However, total daily calcium intake is based on the food product's available calcium rather than its absorption rate.

Supplements are acceptable if you don't get enough calcium in your diet. Calcium citrate and calcium carbonate supplements are equally effective. Calcium citrate can be taken at any time...calcium carbonate should be taken with meals. You can only absorb 500 mg to 600 mg of supplemental calcium at one time. If you're taking more than that, divide it into several daily doses.

• *Don't skip vitamin D.* Most younger adults synthesize adequate vitamin D from the sun, but older adults are less efficient at converting vitamin D into *calcitriol*, the hormone that stimulates calcium absorption.

WHAT MOST PEOPLE DON'T KNOW: If vitamin D levels are low, bone building can be compromised.

Because it can be difficult to get enough of this vitamin, I recommend taking a 400-international unit (IU) supplement of vitamin D daily up to age 65...and 800 IU daily thereafter.

• *Eat vitamin K-rich foods.* Vitamin K helps to aid calcium absorption.

GOOD SOURCES: Red meat, eggs, cereals, fruit (prunes and blueberries) and vegetables (kale and spinach).

CAUTION: Sudden increases in vitamin K intake may decrease the effect of *warfarin* (Coumadin).

WHAT MOST PEOPLE DON'T KNOW: Eating a single daily serving of vitamin K-rich green, leafy vegetables cuts the risk for hip fracture by 50%, compared with eating one serving weekly, according to the landmark Nurses' Health Study.

• *Perform strength training.* In addition to performing weight-bearing exercises, such as walking, running or using the stairs, back-strengthening exercises performed two to three times weekly can significantly increase bone strength.

WHAT MOST PEOPLE DON'T KNOW: Bone responds better to heavier loads than frequent repetitions when weight-lifting.

EXAMPLE: It's better to lift 25 pounds 10 times than to lift five pounds 50 times.

IMPORTANT: If lifestyle measures are not adequate, medications, such as *alendronate* (Fosamax), *raloxifene* (Evista) or *calcitonin-salmon* (Miacalcin), may be needed.

REPORT #93

BUILD BETTER BONES WITH BEER

Source: **Ravin Jugdaohsingh, PhD,** senior research fellow, gastrointestinal laboratory, Rayne Institute, St. Thomas's Hospital, London.

Dietary silicon, which is found in whole grains *and* their products (such as beer), reduces bone loss and promotes bone formation.

Beer is an especially good source of silicon because it is readily absorbed. Other sources of silicon include oat bran, barley and rice.

WARNING: More than two drinks per day for men or one for women is considered harmful.

REPORT #94

SEXUAL HEALING

Source: **Paul Pearsall, PhD,** clinical professor, department of nursing, University of Hawaii at Manoa, and former director of education at the Kinsey Institute at Indiana University, Bloomington. He is author of *A Healing Intimacy* (Three Rivers Press) and *The Pleasure Prescription* (Hunter House).

Sex involves more than procreation—or recreation. As countless studies have shown, an intimate, sexually satisfying relationship reduces the risk of heart disease...depression ...migraine...premenstrual syndrome...and arthritis. It also boosts the immune system.

But sex is genuinely healing *only* if it transcends the mechanical, self-pleasure variety promoted by sex experts.

Indeed, the central goal of sexual healing should not be orgasm—but *connection with your partner*.

PHYSIOLOGY OF HEALING SEX...

Healing sex brings a marked decline in bloodstream levels of *adrenaline* and *cortisol*. These stress hormones provoke anxiety and reduce immune function.

In a study, women who were happily married had higher levels of natural killer cells and helper T cells than those in unhappy unions.

Healing sex is also a potent antidote for social isolation, which has been linked to serious illness and premature death.

A Yale study of 194 heart patients found that those without a spouse at home were twice as likely to die prematurely as those with a spouse.

HEALING SEX IS RARE...

Most couples never experience sexual healing—because they're too quick to give up on their relationship. It takes at least *four years* to achieve the intimacy needed for sexual healing. Most couples split after only three years. Why do so many couples split? Because of lack of intimacy. Intimacy doesn't just happen. You *make* it happen by treating your partner with care and genuine affection...and by taking the time to really connect, both in casual conversation and via sex.

Three factors are central to a sexually healing relationship...

• *Commitment.* Affairs and on-again-off-again sexual relationships are not healing because the two people never form a meaningful bond.

• *Consideration.* The bond between a couple must extend beyond the bedroom. Each partner must continually express tenderness and caring toward the other—by smiling...touching...being polite...giving compliments...and showing respect.

• *Honesty.* There must be no secrets within the relationship—only total connection and total confidence.

HOW TO FORGE A SEXUALLY HEALING RELATIONSHIP...

• *Spend time together.* For at least five minutes a day, sit or lie together—just the two of you. Cuddle. Talk. Let your bodies synchronize.

• *Listen more, talk less.* Ironically, good relationships involve little talk. Partners communicate via their own private language—subtle body movements, gestures, expressions and a sense of connection that arises only between lovers who grow ever closer as a result of sharing crises.

• *Do something special for your partner.* If you spend your days apart, call periodically during the day and say something like, "Honey, I've been thinking about you. I can't wait to see you."

If necessary, set an alarm clock to go off periodically to remind you to place the call.

You come to feel love by behaving lovingly, so even the simplest acts of connection can translate to intense sexual feelings.

• *Have sex only when it feels "right."* Trust your senses. If you rely on your "sex sense" for a month, you'll soon see that when you do have sex, it is more fulfilling and sensual.

• *Seduce your partner.* Instead of dressing up in a sexy costume—as sex therapists often recommend—use "brain power."

Send your partner mental "messages" all day long. At night, lie still in bed and send him/her more "sex waves." You'll be surprised at how seductive your own brain can be.

• *Fantasize about your partner.* Put on some sensual music and lie in bed with your eyes closed. Use your brain—not a vibrator or your hand—and envision yourself making love to your partner.

You may become aroused—even experience orgasm—but mental sex can be surprisingly fulfilling even if you don't.

50-MINUTE SEXUAL FITNESS PLAN...

My sexual fitness plan—which you can add to your weekly exercise regimen—contains three components...

1. Shared laughter. Twenty seconds of laughter produces the same cardiovascular benefits as three minutes of aerobic exercise, studies indicate.

Studies also indicate that a good laugh strengthens the immune system by lowering cortisol levels and raising endorphin levels. And—couples who laugh together become closer and more in tune with one another.

2. Shared crying. Watching a good tearjerker enhances intimacy—and sometimes leads to sexual arousal. Tears, which contain stress hormones and other chemicals, may be nature's way of washing toxins out of the body.

3. Couple "erotorobics." The following suggested sexual exercises may seem strange, but they increase your ability to respond to intimate physical contact...

• Simulated sex. Go through the motions of intercourse—with your clothes on.

• Genital massage. This type of massage stimulates blood flow in that area.

• Dancing to erotic music. Use the muscles you would if you were having intercourse.

• Flirting. Arch your back, sway your hips and stick out your chest. And practice sexual gazing and sexual smiling. Both can make you feel more sensuous.

■

REPORT #95

INCREASE YOUR PLEASURE

Source: **Adriane Fugh-Berman, MD,** assistant clinical professor, department of health care sciences, George Washington University Medical Center, Washington, DC.

Vaginal discomfort in menopause is caused by lower levels of estrogen. It is helped by regular sexual activity, with or without a partner, which promotes circulation and lubrication.

Or—soak a quilted cotton cosmetic square in sesame oil, insert it into the vagina and leave it in overnight, then remove. Repeat daily for a week, then once a week as long as necessary. Vitamin E oil can also be used as a lubricant.

REPORT #96

EAT MORE SOY

Source: **Julian Whitaker, MD,** founder, Whitaker Wellness Institute, Newport Beach, CA, and co-author of *Shed 10 Years in 10 Weeks.* Fireside.

Soy can be sexy for women going through menopause. Soy foods are full of natural plant estrogens. Eating three to four ounces of tofu daily—or drinking one cup of soy milk—can provide an estrogen boost that makes sex more pleasurable.

REPORT #97

MANAGE MENOPAUSE WITHOUT DRUGS

Source: **Toni M. Cutson, MD,** associate professor of community and family medicine and associate professor of medicine, both at Duke University Medical Center in Durham, NC. She is coauthor of "Managing Menopause," a report published in *American Family Physician,* 11400 Tomahawk Creek Pkwy., Leawood, KS 66211.

Hot flashes, mood swings, vaginal dryness, sleep disturbances and other annoying symptoms affect about 75% of menopausal women.

Even more troublesome is the increased risk for heart disease and osteoporosis associated with menopause.

To help control these common problems, doctors in the past prescribed hormone replacement therapy (HRT). Unfortunately, recent evidence suggests that HRT does not protect against heart disease and stroke—in fact, it may increase the risk.

Hormone therapy can also cause side effects, including breast tenderness, bloating and headaches. In addition, it has been linked to a slightly higher risk for breast cancer, especially in women with a family history of the disease.

To avoid the possible drawbacks of HRT, many women treat their symptoms with nondrug alternatives—eating a low-fat, high-fiber diet...exercising regularly...and quitting smoking.

These are a good start. But there are additional ways to relieve the symptoms. Whether she takes hormones or not, a woman can benefit from some commonly overlooked strategies. **THEY INCLUDE...**

• *Eat at least eight servings of fruits and vegetables each day.* These high-fiber, low-fat foods are typically rich in folic acid and other B vitamins, which reduce the risk for heart disease by helping to prevent arterial blood clots.

One serving equals one whole piece of fruit, one-half cup of cooked vegetables or one cup of raw vegetables.

• *Eat whole soy foods.* They contain *isoflavones*, estrogen-like compounds that reduce hot flashes, bone loss and LDL ("bad") cholesterol. Sources include soy nuts, soy milk and tofu.

CAUTION: Avoid any nutritional supplements and powders that claim to have the same active ingredients as soy foods. These products may contain unknown chemicals that could be harmful.

Worse, they may contain *excessive* levels of isoflavones, which increase breast cancer risk. Limit your soy intake to about 60 grams of isoflavones a day.

• *Take a daily multivitamin.* Choose a familiar name brand, such as One-a-Day or Centrum, to make sure you get the recommended requirements for most vitamins and minerals. But do *not* take megadoses of individual vitamins.

Too much vitamin A, for example, can damage the eyes and skin. Megadoses of vitamin D can cause excess calcium in the bloodstream.

To prevent liver damage, avoid pills that provide more than 18 milligrams (mg) of iron. Because menopausal women no longer lose iron through menstruation, iron supplements make sense only if you've been diagnosed with an iron deficiency.

• *Take a calcium supplement.* A daily 1,500-mg dose helps prevent osteoporosis.

Calcium carbonate found in Tums is cheap and readily absorbed. Each Tums tablet provides 500 mg of calcium. For higher doses, try Tums E-X with 750 mg or Tums ULTRA with 1,000 mg.

OSTEOPOROSIS-FIGHTING FOODS: Products that are rich in calcium, such as dairy products (milk and yogurt) and fortified orange juice.

• *Try proven herbal remedies.* Some menopausal women now take chasteberry to prevent hot flashes. But little research exists to support its effectiveness.

Similarly, avoid dong quai and licorice root. Dong quai can cause excessive blood thinning. Licorice root may precipitate headaches or high blood pressure.

BETTER: Black cohosh. This herb suppresses *luteinizing hormone* (LH), which triggers hot flashes. Some women claim it also improves their sex drive and eases night sweats and sleep disturbances.

Black cohosh is sold as Remifemin at health-food stores.

• *Limit alcohol consumption.* Have no more than three glasses of wine—or three ounces of hard liquor—a week. Drinking wine in moderation may be beneficial to the heart, but too much alcohol exacerbates hot flashes.

• *Relax.* Many menopausal women blame hormone fluctuations for their mood and memory problems. But psychological stress is often the real cause. While they're going through menopause, they may also be caring for elderly parents, sending children off to college or dealing with job stress.

TO COMBAT STRESS: Seek help for difficult situations. Turn down extra projects at work...ask siblings to help care for an elderly parent...or find a day program that caters to the social needs of seniors.

Get plenty of sleep and give yourself 30 minutes of quiet time each day. If your schedule doesn't permit it, five minutes is better than nothing.

• *Rethink your sex life.* The physical and psychological aspects of menopause often put a damper on a woman's sex life. But abstinence is not the answer.

Frequent sexual activity decreases vaginal dryness, improves sleep, reduces stress and helps alleviate moodiness.

BONUS: Regular sex also increases your libido.

■

REPORT #98

BEYOND BLACK COHOSH: SMARTER SOLUTIONS FOR MENOPAUSE

Source: **Mark A. Stengler, ND,** naturopathic physician in private practice, La Jolla, CA…associate clinical professor at the National College of Naturopathic Medicine, Portland, OR…author of numerous books, including *The Natural Physician's Healing Therapies* and coauthor of *Prescription for Natural Cures* (both from Bottom Line Books)…and author of the *Bottom Line/Natural Healing* newsletter.

Nearly 38 million American women are between the ages of 40 and 54, according to the US Census Bureau. They all are in some stage of menopause. If you're among them, I'm sure you're wondering about the best ways to deal with the symptoms. Fortunately, several natural remedies and medicines can help. They are safe and effective—and some work quickly, particularly if you have mild to moderate symptoms.

Menopause is a normal stage in a woman's life. Once a woman hasn't had a period for 12 consecutive months, she has reached menopause. In the US, the average age is 51. During menopause, ovaries produce less of the hormones estrogen, progesterone and testosterone.

Meanwhile, there's an increase in the release of two hormones produced by the pituitary gland—*follicle stimulating hormone* (FSH) and *luteinizing hormone.* Doctors believe the surge of these hormones triggers menopausal symptoms, including hot flashes (which affect three-quarters of American menopausal women) and vaginal dryness. You also may experience insomnia, depression and mood swings.

In the year or two before menopause starts, many women go through perimenopause, or premenopause, during which hot flashes and other symptoms usually begin. The menstrual cycle becomes irregular. A period of lingering symptoms *after* menopause is called postmenopause. The therapies I recommend are effective for women in any stage, from perimenopause to postmenopause—but not one of these therapies includes typical pharmaceuticals. **HERE'S WHY...**

THE HORMONE HERESY...

Sixty years ago, doctors started giving women synthetic estrogen along with a synthetic form of progesterone known as *progestin* to control menopausal symptoms. Premarin, one of these formulas, has been one of the best-selling drugs in recent history—but I view it as one of the biggest scams of all time.

Premarin, and drugs like it, were said to offer many benefits, including prolonged youthfulness, a sound mind, improved libido, strong bones and a healthy heart. I never believed the hype, nor did many other preventive-medicine doctors.

The dangers of taking hormone formulas came to light a few years ago. Doctors and female patients were alarmed at the results of a study on the drug Prempro, a combination of Premarin and a synthetic progesterone called Provera. Prempro had been touted as a panacea for menopausal problems, but views changed in July 2002, when results of the Women's Health Initiative Study, which included more than 16,000 women, showed unexpected dangers from the drug. Investigators found significant increases in risk of heart disease, stroke, blood clots and breast cancer among women taking Prempro.

In 2003, the Women's Health Initiative Memory Study revealed that women 65 and older who had been taking Prempro had an increased risk of dementia. Premarin has been shown to increase gallbladder disease risk.

Additionally, the British Million Women Study found that the use of hormone replacement therapy by women ages 50 to 64 over the past decade had resulted in an estimated 20,000 additional breast cancers and an increased incidence of fatal breast malignancies.

The response of pharmaceutical giants makes my hair stand on end—they recommended lower dosages of the drugs, even though there were no studies showing that lower

doses were safer. Companies also started promoting pharmaceutical antidepressants, such as *venlafaxine* (Effexor),
fluoxetine (Prozac), *paroxetine* (Paxil) and *sertraline* (Zoloft),
for relief of menopausal symptoms, especially hot flashes. All
these drugs have potential side effects—including fatigue,
headache, worsening of depression and weight gain.

Fortunately, many natural therapies are readily available.
Natural therapy's goal is to alleviate or reduce symptoms
quickly without harmful side effects. I recommend starting
with nutritional supplements—including various herbal and
homeopathic therapies.

MILD TO MODERATE SYMPTOMS...

Women with "mild" symptoms may be annoyed by occasional hot flashes. Those in the "moderate" category have hot
flashes along with other symptoms. For example, if a woman
experiences three or four hot flashes a day, doesn't sleep at
night and has reduced sex drive, I consider her symptoms to
be moderate. You can take these remedies one at a time or
use a formula that contains some or all of the ingredients.

• *Black cohosh.* This shrub was used by Native Americans
for hormonal problems. At least six studies have shown that it
can help relieve hot flashes, night sweats and depression. One
popular brand of black cohosh is Remifemin, which is available at pharmacies and at Drugstore.com. Choose an extract
standardized to 2.5% *triterpene glycosides* (an ingredient that
helps control luteinizing hormone). Start by taking a dose of
80 milligrams (mg) daily and increase to 160 mg daily if necessary. Many women notice improvement within two to four
weeks. You can take black cohosh for four to six months, then
stop to see if your symptoms return. If they do, resume taking it. In rare cases, black cohosh can cause digestive upset,
headache and/or dizziness.

• *Vitex (chasteberry).* This hormone-regulating herb has
been recommended since the days of Hippocrates. Use vitex during perimenopause to reduce heavy bleeding and hot
flashes. Take 160 mg to 240 mg of a 0.6% *aucubin* standardized extract or 40 drops of the tincture daily. The company
Vitanica (800-572-4712, *www.vitanica.com*) offers a 0.6% aucubin extract, which is available at health-food stores. You

can take it for as long as you have symptoms. Vitex should not be taken with birth control pills.

HOMEOPATHIC FORMULAS...

Work with a practitioner trained in homeopathy who can match your symptoms to appropriate compounds. The following remedies are available at most health-food stores. For each, start with two pellets of a 30C potency twice daily. You should notice positive results within two weeks. After symptoms improve, stop taking the remedy unless symptoms return.

• *Sepia* helps with hot flashes, night sweats and vaginal dryness. It is recommended for women who feel short-tempered, irritable, have a low libido or when symptoms include incontinence or uterine prolapse (falling or sliding of the uterus from its normal position in the pelvic cavity into the vaginal canal).

• *Lachesis* is good for hot flashes, anxiety, headaches, insomnia, heart palpitations and irritability.

• *Pulsatilla* is for women who feel much worse in a warm room. It also is recommended if you have mood swings, weepiness or a strong craving for sweets.

• *Sulphur* helps relieve insomnia and is excellent for women who are constantly overheated, sweat easily and have a strong thirst for ice-cold drinks.

MODERATE TO SEVERE SYMPTOMS...

• *Natural progesterone cream* is helpful for women with stronger symptoms. I advise perimenopausal women to apply 20 mg of the cream (about one-quarter teaspoon) on the inside of their wrists and forearms or other areas of the body one to two times daily for the last two weeks of their menstrual cycles. Do not use it during your period. If you're menopausal, apply the same amount one to two times daily. Stop using it five to seven days each month unless your symptoms return during this time. Postmenopausal women should apply 10 mg (about one-eighth teaspoon) one to two times daily, again with five to seven days off each month.

VISIT YOUR DOCTOR FIRST...

Before taking anything for menopausal symptoms, see your family doctor or gynecologist. I recommend at least a yearly visit. In addition to having a complete physical (including a

Pap smear test and a bone scan), ask your doctor about a comprehensive saliva hormone assessment. The doctor collects saliva samples and sends them to a lab to determine hormone balance and identify deficiencies. This method is accurate and cost-effective. One good saliva hormone testing lab is ZRT Laboratory (503-466-2445, *www.salivatest.com*). Testing can cost $150 to $240 and may be covered by insurance.

For a referral to a doctor who is knowledgeable about natural hormone testing, contact...

• *The American Association of Naturopathic Physicians,* 866-538-2267, *www.naturopathic.org.*

• *American College for Advancement in Medicine,* 800-532-3688, *www.acam.org.*

■

REPORT #99

UNCOMMON CURES FOR EVERYDAY COMPLAINTS

Source: **Larry Altshuler, MD,** founder and medical director, Balanced Healing Medical Center, Oklahoma City (*www.balancedhealing.com*), and author of *Bottom Line's Balanced Healing.* Bottom Line Books.

Even though numerous major medical centers have begun combining alternative healing techniques with conventional medical therapies, most medical doctors in private practice still don't recommend these approaches to their patients. That's because most MDs aren't familiar enough with alternative medicine to know what works and what doesn't.

Here are four underused alternative therapies you may want to try*...

ACUPUNCTURE...

In the US, acupuncture is used primarily to treat chronic pain and various addictions. The procedure is believed to stimulate the different types of nerves that activate parts of

*Before trying any of these treatments, consult your physician to ensure that they do not interfere with any other therapy you are receiving.

the brain involved in healing and in the transmission and perception of pain.

Each acupuncture session typically requires the insertion of eight to 12 needles, which usually penetrate the skin one to one-and-a-half inches. The procedure causes little to no pain. And, symptoms generally diminish within just six sessions.

Conditions that often improve with acupuncture treatments...

• *Asthma.* Prescription inhalers and medication are the first-line treatment for asthma—but adding acupuncture treatments usually helps to reduce the severity and the frequency of future attacks. In some instances, the use of acupuncture enables patients to decrease their asthma medication.

• *Depression.* Acupuncture is believed to rebalance the brain neurotransmitters that are involved in depression.

In our clinic, we usually begin by prescribing acupuncture along with ongoing psychotherapy and natural antidepressants, such as St. John's wort—300 milligrams (mg) daily...ginkgo biloba—160 to 240 mg daily...and/or fish oil—4 grams (g) daily.

If there's still no improvement in the patient's depression, we then prescribe antidepressant medication.

• *Hay fever.* Acupuncture is the fastest and most effective way I have found to reduce or eliminate respiratory allergies. Most people can discontinue their medications following acupuncture treatment.

• *Migraines.* Acupuncture is one of the best treatments for an acute migraine attack, typically relieving pain within 30 minutes.

Each subsequent session also decreases the frequency and severity of attacks and may even cure them completely.

With their doctor's consent, most people can discontinue their medication, although some will still take it for occasional headaches or if they can't get in to see an acupuncturist.

• *Smoking.* Almost 80% of people can stop smoking with the help of acupuncture, according to studies.

If you try acupuncture, consult a practitioner trained in traditional Chinese acupuncture and certified by the National Certification Commission for Acupuncture and Oriental Medicine (703-548-9004, *www.nccaom.org*).

CRANIAL–SACRAL MANIPULATION...

This technique, which is administered by a doctor of osteopathy (DO), involves manipulating the bones in the face and skull. It helps correct misalignments caused by obstructions, overloaded muscles and joints, and other structural problems in various parts of the spine.

Symptoms typically diminish with three to six treatments.

Conditions that often improve with cranial–sacral manipulation…

• *Sinus problems.* Sinusitis brought on by a structural obstruction responds well to this type of treatment.

• *Temporomandibular joint (TMJ) syndrome.* Manipulation can be useful to ease the headaches associated with this misalignment of the TMJ, which connects the jawbone to the skull—especially when the misalignment results from an accident.

• *Tinnitus (ringing in the ears).* Manipulation helps to correct structural abnormalities in the bones surrounding the ear, which can lead to tinnitus.

If you want to try cranial–sacral manipulation, consult an osteopathic physician certified by the American Osteopathic Association (800-621-1773, *www.osteopathic.org*).

HYPNOSIS…

In this mind–body technique, the hypnotist places you in a deeply relaxed state and makes positive suggestions regarding your emotions, habits and bodily functions. Symptoms typically diminish with two to three sessions.

Conditions that often improve with hypnosis treatments…

• *Anxiety and phobias.* In the cases where psychotherapy brings no improvement, hypnosis is often effective.

• *Chronic pain.* Hypnosis can decrease ongoing pain by addressing emotional and psychological triggers.

• *Irritable bowel syndrome (IBS).* Persistent IBS frequently has underlying psychological causes, which quite often can be alleviated through hypnosis. One study discovered that hypnosis therapy alleviated the symptoms in 90% of IBS sufferers.

• *Overeating.* Hypnotic suggestion can help curb the urge to eat between meals and reduce the desire to eat unhealthy foods.

If you try hypnosis, consult with a hypnotist belonging to the American Society of Clinical Hypnosis (630-980-4740, *www.asch.net*) or to the National Guild of Hypnotists (603-429-9438, *www.ngh.net*).

MASSAGE...

Massage boosts levels of the feel-good neurotransmitter known as *serotonin* while lowering levels of stress hormones.

Two commonly used types of massage are Swedish massage (which uses gentle pressure and broad stroking movements to help relax the muscles) or shiatsu massage (in which finger pressure is placed on key healing points along the body).

Symptoms typically begin to diminish after the person receives the first massage.

Conditions that frequently improve with massage therapy...

• *Anxiety.* Massage is an excellent treatment for reducing mild anxiety states. It has been shown to reduce or block the effects of *cortisol* and *epinephrine*, hormones that can damage body tissue when they are produced at excessive levels during anxiety-provoking or stressful conditions.

• *Back problems.* Massage will provide the most relief when it's used in conjunction with over-the-counter *nonsteroidal anti-inflammatory drugs* (NSAIDs), hot/cold compresses and/ or ultrasound treatment, which incorporates high-frequency sound (20,000 Hz) and heat.

• *Tension headaches.* Pressure applied to trigger points in the neck, forehead and temples relieves most tension headaches.

Thirty-six states now license massage therapists. To find one, contact the American Massage Therapy Association at 877-905-2700 or *www.amtamassage.org.*

You also can ask your doctor for a referral.

■

REPORT #100

READ THIS NOW TO GROW
15 YEARS YOUNGER

Source: **Michael F. Roizen, MD,** chief of the division of anesthesiology, critical care medicine and comprehensive pain management at the Cleveland Clinic. He is author of *RealAge* and *The RealAge Makeover* (both from HarperCollins). He is founder of RealAge.com, where you can calculate your own RealAge.

How old are you really? We all have a "real age" that can be much lower—or higher—than our chronological years. A

50-year-old man, for example, could have the immune system of someone 20 years younger.

More than a decade ago, I introduced the RealAge concept —a scientific way of calculating a number that reflects the overall state of your health rather than your calendar age. We are constantly updating our data to reflect new research. The lower your RealAge, the longer you are likely to live.

We discovered that some changes can be hard to achieve— such as losing 25 pounds or quitting smoking—but others are relatively easy and can have a big impact on your life span.

LATEST FINDINGS: Recent research pinpoints 10 simple changes that can lower your RealAge by almost 15 years...

TAKE ASPIRIN DAILY...

REALAGE BENEFIT: 2.2 years

In men over age 35 and women over age 40, 162 milli-grams (mg) of aspirin daily (the equivalent of two baby as-pirins) reduces the risk of heart attack by 36% and the risk of colon, esophageal, throat and stomach cancers by about 40%. We don't know how aspirin reduces cancer risk—we just know that it does.

Check with your doctor about taking aspirin. Some people can't take it because of allergies, stomach discomfort and/or bleeding. Ibuprofen may be an appropriate substitute.

CAUTION: Taking both aspirin and ibuprofen in the same 24-hour period blocks the protective effects. Also, don't take aspirin in combination with blood-thinning drugs such as *warfarin* (Coumadin). It increases the risk of internal bleeding.

SUPPLEMENT WITH FOLATE...

REALAGE BENEFIT: 1.2 years

The B vitamin folate helps prevent errors in DNA duplica-tion, an underlying cause of cancer. Taking 600 micrograms (mcg) to 800 mcg of folate daily could decrease breast cancer risk by 25% to 50%...colon cancer risk by 20% to 50%...and risk of childhood cancers by about 60% when taken by the mother during pregnancy. Folate also lowers levels of *homo-cysteine*, an amino acid linked to stroke, heart disease and other cardiovascular disorders.

Take a B-complex or multisupplement that includes 100%
of the recommended daily amount of the vitamins B-6 and B-
12...and add a folate supplement to get a total of 600 to 800
mcg daily. You need all three to lower homocysteine—and the
ability of the body to absorb B-12 declines with age.

DON'T SUPPLEMENT UNNECESSARILY...

REALAGE BENEFIT: 1.7 years

Millions of Americans take iron or vitamin A supplements
daily. With the exception of some people who, for specific reasons, are advised by their doctors to take extra vitamin A or
extra iron, the use of these nutrients (except in a multivitamin) can take years off your life.

The average vitamin A supplement contains more than 5,000
international units (IU), an amount that causes bone deminer-
alization and increases the risk of liver and lung cancers.

Taking iron is dangerous because as many as one in 200
Americans has hemochromatosis, a condition that causes excess iron to accumulate in tissues, increasing the risk of heart
or liver failure.

I advise taking a daily multivitamin that contains all the
essential vitamins and minerals but no iron unless told to by
your doctor. The multivitamin should contain less than 2,500
IU of vitamin A.

EAT SPAGHETTI SAUCE...

REALAGE BENEFIT: 1.9 years for men, 0.8 years for women.

Tomatoes contain the carotenoid *lycopene*, which is believed to strengthen the immune system and reduce the risk
of breast and prostate cancers by 30% to 50%. Try to get 10
tablespoons (a little more than one-half cup) of tomato sauce
weekly. Processed tomatoes, such as those in spaghetti sauce,
confer more benefits than fresh tomatoes because processing
releases the lycopene. Eat canned tomatoes or tomato sauce
with a little oil—for example, by cooking the sauce with olive
oil—to improve absorption of lycopene.

CONSUME FAT FIRST AT MEALS...

REALAGE BENEFIT: 1.8 years.

Starting meals with a little fat increases feelings of satiety
and reduces overall calorie intake by about 7%. If you are

overweight, you can lose about 10 pounds in a year if you do this at every meal.

Make sure that the fat is a healthy one—olive oil, nuts, etc. To get the benefits, you need about 70 calories of fat, which is about one-half tablespoon of olive oil, six walnuts or 12 almonds. One great way to start a meal is with a salad that has olive oil in the dressing and a few chopped nuts sprinkled on top.

WASH PRODUCE—AND YOUR HANDS...

REALAGE BENEFIT: 0.4 years.

More than 40 million Americans suffer from food poisoning annually, and several thousand die from foodborne illness. Washing your hands frequently—and always before meals—is a key way to prevent this.

It's also crucial to wash produce thoroughly. Even organic fruits and vegetables require washing because they contain fertilizer residue that can cause illness. Wash produce twice in lukewarm water with a little dish soap, then rinse twice in regular water. You can put greens in a salad spinner and give them three cycles of rinsing/spinning.

DRINK MODERATELY...

REALAGE BENEFIT: 1.9 years.

Alcohol reduces the tendency of blood platelets to clump together and form clots in the arteries, the cause of most heart attacks. It also inhibits the oxidation of fat that contributes to the development of plaque on artery walls.

The extensive Harvard Nurses' Health Study found that women who had three or more alcoholic drinks weekly had a 40% lower rate of heart attacks and arterial disease than those who did not. Studies in men show similar results.

CAUTION: Moderation is the key—one-half to one drink daily for women, and one to two drinks daily for men. Don't drink alcohol if you have a history of drug or alcohol abuse.

GET ENOUGH SUN...

REALAGE BENEFIT: 1.7 years.

Vitamin D is essential for calcium absorption and bone strength. It also helps reduce the risk of breast, colon, prostate and lung cancers. Only a few foods (mainly fatty fish) contain vitamin D in a form that can be used by the body. Sunshine is required to convert fats in the body into a usable form of vitamin D.

I advise getting 10 to 20 minutes of daily sun exposure without using sunscreen. Use sunscreen when you're in the sun longer than 20 minutes to prevent premature skin aging and skin cancer.

EAT FIBER EARLY IN THE DAY...

REALAGE BENEFIT: 0.6 years.

Starting the day with a high-fiber cereal or fresh fruits or vegetables helps you feel full longer and reduces calorie intake. It prevents spikes in glucose that can damage arteries and increase the risk of heart disease.

BONUS: People who get at least 25 grams of fiber a day have a RealAge up to three years younger than those who get the national average of 12 grams.

EXAMPLE: In a study recently conducted at Northwestern University, a 10-gram-a-day increase in cereal fiber consumption decreased the risk of heart attack by 29%.